AAS
Agents and Actions Supplements
Vol. 35

Series Editor
K. Brune, Erlangen

Birkhäuser Verlag
Basel · Boston · Berlin

Progress in Inflammation Research and Therapy

Based on the Fifth International Conference of the Inflammation Research Association, September 23–27, 1990, White Haven, PA, USA

Edited by

N. R. Ackerman
R. J. Bonney
A. F. Welton

Birkhäuser Verlag
Basel · Boston · Berlin

Volume Editors' Addresses:

Dr. N. R. Ackerman
Glycomed, Inc.
860 Atlantic Avenue
Alameda, CA 94501
USA

Dr. R. J. Bonney
Bristol-Myers Squibb
Pharmaceutical Res. Inst.
100 Forest Avenue
Buffalo, NY 14213
USA

Dr. A. F. Welton
Hoffmann-La Roche Inc.
340 Kingsland St.
Nutley, NJ 07110
USA

Library of Congress Cataloging-in-Publication Data

Inflammation Research Association. International Conference (5th : 1990 : White Haven, Pa.)
Progress in inflammation research and therapy : based on the Fifth International Conference of the Inflammation Research Association, September 23-27, 1990, White Haven, PA, USA. / edited by N. R. Ackerman, R. J. Bonney, A. F. Welton.
(Agents and actions supplements ; vol. 35)
Includes bibliographical references.
ISBN 3-7643-2529-1 (acid-free paper) – ISBN 0-8176-2529-1 (acid-free paper)
1. Inflammation-Congresses. 2. Inflammation-Mediators-Congresses. 3. Anti-inflammatory agents-Congresses.
I. Ackerman, Neil. II. Bonney, R. J. (Robert J.), 1942– .
III. Welton, A. F. (Ann F.), 1947– . IV. Title. V. Series:
Agents and actions supplements ; AAS 35.
[DNLM: 1. Anti-Inflammatory Agents-therapeutic use-congresses.
2. Inflammation-drug therapy-congresses. W1 AG33A v. 35 / QV 247 I43p 1990]
RB131.I 545 1990 616'.0473 – dc20

Deutsche Bibliothek Cataloging-in-Publication Data

Progress in inflammation research and therapy: based on the 5. International Conference of the Inflammation Research Association, September 23–27, 1990, White Haven, PA, USA / ed. by N. R. Ackerman ... – Basel ; Boston ; Berlin : Birkhäuser, 1991
(Agents and actions : Supplements ; Vol. 35)
ISBN 3-7643-2529-1 (Basel ...)
ISBN 0-8176-2529-1 (Boston)
NE: Ackerman, Neil R. [Hrsg.]; Agents and actions / Supplements

Printed in Germany on acid-free paper
ISBN 3-7643-2529-1
ISBN 0-8176-2529-1

Contents

Workshop Sessions

Poster Discussion

Preface

The Inflammation Research Association was founded in 1970 with the objectives of reviewing current approaches and therapies for inflammatory diseases. Investigators researching these diseases in the 1970's and 80's had as their major findings the role of various arachidonic acid products in the pathogenesis of inflammation. From the therapeutic perspective, the early 1970's were of major importance for the introduction of the non-steroidal anti-inflammatory drugs. Indomethacin and phenylbutazone were amongst the first to be introduced; these were improved upon with agents having a longer duration of action and/or a better safety profile. The most prescribed agents naproxen (Naprosyn), piroxicam (Feldene) and diclofenac (Voltaren) were introduced over the following twenty years.

All of these agents are thought to function primarily via their ability to inhibit the enzyme prostaglandin synthetase thereby interfering with the generation of prostaglandins, especially of the E class. No other anti-inflammatory drugs have reached the marketplace having a profile different from that of the classical non-steroidal agents. A great deal of information however, has been generated over the last two decades which provides the basis for complementary therapeutic agents. Of most importance is the role of the leukotrienes in many inflammation-based diseases such as rheumatoid arthritis, ulcerative colitis and psoriasis. Similarly the cytokines, especially interleukin 1, have been implicated in the pathogenesis of these same disease states. At present two agents, the Abbott Laboratories 5 lipoxygenase inhibitor A-64077, and Synergen's interleukin 1 receptor antagonist, are the most promising in a series of new anti-inflammatory drugs functioning via these newer mechanisms. Both are in a clinical studies with efficacy results expected within one-two years.

In addition to the leukotriene and cytokine-based approaches many other strategies are available to researchers studying inflammatory diseases. These include influencing the proteinases involved in connective tissue breakdown, blocking adhesion required for the infiltration of leukocytes and selectively inhibiting the underlying immunologic defects leading to an inflammatory cascade. One or more of these approaches may serve to provide therapeutics having important clinical benefits in the years to come.

History of the Inflammation Research Association

The Inflammation Research Association (IRA) was founded in 1970 by a group of scientists from east coast pharmaceutical companies in the USA as a forum for discussion of methodologies used in inflammation research. It quickly expanded its horizons to cover the design and discovery of new and improved therapies for inflammatory diseases and attracted a wider audience. C. Gordon van Arman, Marvin Rosethale, Ed Takesue, and Mary Lee Graeme were largely responsible for the initiation of the IRA, and set many of the unwritten ground rules for the Association.

The organization of the IRA has evolved over the years. Initially it consisted of only a President and Treasurer, but the organization was expanded in 1984 to include additional board members. This more formal structure was necessitated by the success of the First and Second International Conferences of the IRA that were held in November, 1982 and October, 1984, respectively. The local and overseas support of these conferences and the large number of people willing to take an active organizational role, allowed the IRA to reach the status of a national organization. The Third and Fourth International Conferences were held in October, 1986 and October, 1988, respectively and were attended by investigators from many nations, making the term "International Conference"* a reality. The Fifth Conference in this series was held in September, 1990 and the proceedings are contained in this book.

In addition to the scientific sessions, workshops and poster presentations, the IRA, during the Fourth International Conference,

*Adapted from Therapeutic Approaches to Inflammatory Diseases, edited by A. J. Lewis, N. S. Doherty and N. R. Ackerman, Elsevier Science Publishing Co., Inc. 1989 p.x.

sponsored C. Gordon van Arman Awards to recognize research in inflammation among graduate students and postdoctoral fellows. Dr. van Arman has had a long and illustrious research career as an industrial scientist and has been a long standing member of the IRA. By establishing this award, the IRA acknowledges these accomplishments, his enthusiasm for inflammation research and his encouragement of young scientists. In this Fifth Conference poster discussions were held for the first time. In these sessions the poster presenters provided brief overviews of their research for an audience consisting primarily of specialists in their respective technologies.

The increase in attendees with each successive conference suggests that an important need is being met by the IRA. The membership now approximates 1500 and has a high percentage of industrial members. The Association has been headed by industrial scientists from the beginning (see Table I) and as a result, the flavor and

Table 1. IRA Officers (1970 – Present)

Year	*President*	*Treasurer*	*Secretary*
1970	Ed Takesue *Sandoz*	—	—
1972	Marvin Rosenthale *Wyeth*	C. Gordon van Arman *Merck & Co.*	Mary Lee Graeme *CIBA-GEIGY*
1975	Duane Sofia *Carter Wallace*	Stewart Wong *McNeil*	—
1978	Lawerence Sancilio *A. H. Robins*	Stewart Wong *McNeil*	—
1980	Stewart Wong *Boehringer-Ingelheim*	Robert Capetola *Ortho*	—
1982	Robert Capetola *Ortho*	Ivan Otterness *Pfizer*	—
1984	Ivan Otterness *Pfizer*	Alan Lewis *Wyeth*	Lian Liauw *CIBA-GEIGY*
1986	Alan Lewis *Wyeth-Ayerst*	Neil Ackerman *DuPont*	Lian Liauw *CIBA-GEIGY*
1988	Neil Ackerman *DuPont*	Robert Bonney *Bristol-Myers*	Marcia Bliven *Pfizer*
1990	Robert Bonney *Bristol-Myers Squibb*	Niall Doherty *Pfizer*	Joan Chapdelaine *Pharmakon*

direction of both the monthly and international meetings is focused on the scientific basis, design, development and clinical testing of new therapies for inflammatory and immunologically mediated diseases.

Committee Members

Planning

Neil R. Ackerman
Marcia L. Bliven
Robert J. Bonney

Advertising

Janet S. Kerr

Audio-Visual

Thomas J. Carty, Chairperson
Elaine M. Bruin
Ann Cunningham
Ronald Laliberte
Linda Tomchek

Finance

Barry M. Weichman, Conference Treasurer

On-Site Registration

Theresa M. Stevens, Chairperson
Lisa R. Mantegna

Poster Session

Thomas B. Stim, Chairperson
William E. Hageman, Chairperson

Poster Discussion

Kathleen R. Gans-Brangs, Chairperson
Richard B. Gibertsen

Richard R. Harris
Janet S. Kerr
Lisa A. Marshall
Douglas W. Morgan
Nigel D. Staite
Kenneth M. Tramposch
Barry M. Weichman

Professional Advancement

William E. Hageman, Chairperson

Publications
Book (Editors)

Neil R. Ackerman
Robert J. Bonney
Ann F. Welton

Mini-Papers

Niall S. Doherty

Registrar

Joan M. Chapdelaine

Scientific Program

Robert J. Bonney, Chairperson
Daniel E. Furst
John L. Humes
Leland Loose
William M. Mackin
Martha R. Matteo
Robert C. Thompson
Daniel E. Tracey
Joseph C. Williams

Scholarship

Richard P. Carlson, Co-Chairperson
Alan J. Lewis, Co-Chairperson
Michael J. DiMartino
Richard B. Gilbertsen
John L. Humes
Ivan G. Otterness
Robert J. Smith

Site Coordination/Travel Arrangements

H. Lian Liauw, Chairperson
Marcia L. Bliven
Richard P. Carlson
Thomas B. Stim
Deborah A. Wolff

Social Events

Gary Peterman, Chairperson

Workshop Sessions

Ann F. Welton, Chairperson
Richard P. Carlson
George W. Carter
Ronald L. Goldberg
Joanne T. Hom
L. Gordon Letts
Alan J. Lewis
David Y. Liu
Rodger M. McMillan
Margaret O'Donnell
Adrian N. Payne
Edith R. Schwartz
Philip J. Simon
James E. Talmadge
Daniel R. Twardzic

Acknowledgements

The manuscripts contained in this volume are based on material presented at the Fifth International Conference of the Inflammation Research Association held in White Haven, Pennsylvania, on September 23–27, 1990.

We would like to thank the speakers and session chairpersons for their major contributions to the conference and this Proceeding. A listing of all Committee Members is presented on the next page.

The generous financial support of the following companies is greatly appreciated:

Abbott Laboratories, Allergan Pharmaceuticals, Inc., Biomol Research Labs, Inc., Boehringer-Ingelheim Pharmaceuticals, Inc., Bristol-Myers Squibb Company, Burroughs Wellcome Company, CIBA-GEIGY Corporation, Cytogen Corporation, E.I. du Pont de Nemours & Company, Inc., Genentech, Inc., Glaxo, Inc., Hoffmann-La Roche Inc., ICI Pharmaceuticals Group, The R. W. Johnson Pharmaceutical Research Institute, Lilly Research Laboratories, Merck-Frosst Canada, Inc., Merck Sharp & Dohme Research Laboratories, Merrell Dow Research Institute of Marion Merrell Dow Inc., Miles Inc./Bayer AG, Parke-Davis Pharmaceuticals Research, Division of Warner Lambert, Pfizer Central Research, Pharmacon Research International, Inc., Riker Labs, Inc./3M Company, Schering-Plough Research, G.D. Searle & Company, SmithKline Beecham Pharmaceuticals, Sterling Drug, Inc., Synergen, Inc., Syntex Research, The Upjohn Company, Wyeth-Ayerst Research.

Plenary Presentation

AAS 35
Progress in Inflammation
Research and Therapy

Molecular Mechanisms of Leukocyte Activation by Chemoattractants

R. Snyderman and J. Didsbury

Department of Medicine, Duke University Medical Center, Box 3680, Durham, NC 27710, USA

Summary

Chemoattractant receptors on leukocytes initiate migratory and cytotoxic activities via GTP-binding proteins. Recent cloning of cDNA encoding the formylpeptide receptor indicates it to be a member of the class of seven membrane spanning domain receptors which couple to G proteins. Leukocyte activation by chemoattractants requires sequential metabolic pathways involving phospholipase C then phospholipase D. Interestingly, the formylpeptide receptor physically associates with both a heterotrimeric G protein and a low molecular mass GTP-binding protein. These multiple GTP-binding proteins may regulate the function of chemoattractant receptors.

The ability of phagocytic leukocytes (polymorphonuclear leukocytes and macrophages) to accumulate and become activated at sites of inflammatory reactions is a prerequisite for their functioning in host defence. Phagocytes migrate along gradients of chemoattractants produced by humoral and cellular immune responses. Defined chemotactic factors include C5a, a complement proteolytic fragment, leukotriene B_4 (LTB_4), an arachidonate metabolite, platelet-activating factor (PAF) and certain products of bacterial protein synthesis (i.e. formylmethionyl peptides). N-formylated synthetic oligopeptides [e.g. N-formyl-methionyl-leucyl phenyalanine, (fMet-Leu-Phe or fMLP)] which are similar to these products are useful probes to study leukocyte activation (Synderman et al., 1990).

The response of leukocytes to chemoattractants is initiated by ligation of cell surface receptors. Specific receptors for chemotactic factors are present on phagocytic leukocytes and when activated initiate a cascade of events which lead to the localization of phagocytes at sites of inflammation and the activation of their cytotoxic potential. The best characterized chemotactic factor receptor is the one which binds formylpeptides. While much is known about this receptor the precise mechanics by which chemoattractant receptors initiate migratory versus cytotoxic activities remains to be determined. Recent advances in this field now make it possible to identify the structure-function relationships of chemoattractant receptors for their activation of disparate cellular functions.

Chemoattractants not only stimulate the directed migration of leukocytes but also may induce them to secrete lysosomal enzymes and produce superoxide anions. Interestingly, motility-related functions occur at low doses of chemoattractants (ca. 10^{-9} M fMLP) whereas secretory functions require 20–50-fold higher concentrations (Synderman et al., 1988). Both of these responses are initiated by binding of chemoattractants to specific cell surface receptors.

In addition to their location on the cell surface, formylpeptide receptors cosediment with specific granule membranes suggesting that an intracellular pool of receptors may be available for recruitment to the cell surface (Jesaitis et al., 1982). Indeed after fMLP binding, the number of cell surface receptors increases and receptors internalize suggesting receptor recycling.

Neutrophil receptors for both lipid (LTB_4, PAF) and peptide (C5a, fMLP) chemoattractants all possess a single ligand binding subunit and appear to be monomeric (for review see Snyderman et al., 1990). The molecular mass of fMLP, C5a and LTB_4 receptors is similar with kDas of $\sim$50–70. The total number of receptors for each chemoattractant is in the same moderately abundant range with $0.5–2.8 \times 10^5$ receptors per cell. Two classes of binding sites, one high affinity (Kd 0.2–0.5 nM) and one low affinity (Kd 20–500 nM) are found for each receptor. Guanine nucleotides modulate the interconvertibility of high affinity to low affinity sites for each of these receptors suggesting that each chemoattractant receptor is associated with a G protein. Based on these similarities it is likely that all of these receptors will be structurally homologous to one another and like other G protein-coupled receptors will contain a seven membrane spanning domain structure with extracellular and cytoplasmic tails. Indeed, the recent cloning of the formylpeptide receptor (Boulay et al., 1990) has shown it to possess this structure, characteristic of G protein-coupled receptors.

In addition to the above mentioned properties of the formylpeptide receptor, several other lines of evidence demonstrate its association with G proteins (Synderman et al., 1988). Prebound formylpeptide receptor-ligand complexes on intact permeabilized neutrophils undergo an increased rate of dissociation in response to GTPγS and a partially purified formylpeptide receptor-radioligand complex exhibited a similar response to GTPγS. Our laboratory has also shown that the formylpeptide receptor-radioligand complex elutes in three distinct peaks when chromatographed on DEAE-Fractogel. One peak is free receptor, a second co-elutes with a 40 kDa pertussis toxin substrate which we have identified as Giα2. Interestingly, a third peak of receptor is associated with a ca. 28 kDa GTP-binding protein (Polakis et al., 1989). Both the 40 kDa G protein and the low molecular mass GTP-binding protein are physically associated with the receptor since GTPγS enhances ligand dissociation from the complex and dissociation of the receptor from the GTP-binding proteins. Furthermore, fMLP stimulates both GTPase activity and the rate of GTPγS binding to leukocyte membranes.

These results imply association of the formylpeptide receptor with multiple G proteins and a potential role for low molecular mass G proteins in signal transduction or transport of the receptor to the cell surface. The low molecular mass G proteins appear to be involved in a broad array of cell functions including differentiation, growth, cytoskeletal organization and vesicular transport and secretion (Hall, 1990).

Neutrophil responses to chemoattractants fall into two broad types and recognition of this phenomenon is proving useful in delineating the biochemical mechanisms which govern the migratory versus cytotoxic (microbicidal/secretory) activities of the cells (Snyderman et al., 1988, 1990). The evidence for discrete regulation of the two types of responses are based on dose-response relationships, activity of different chemoattractants, kinetics and pharmacological manipulations. Migratory or chemotactic responses occur at doses of chemoattractant which are at least 20-fold lower than those needed to stimulate cytotoxic processes such as the respiratory burst or exocytosis. Based on our biochemical studies the mechanism of phagocyte activation by the chemoattractant fMet-Leu-Phe can be put into the framework of two sequential phases. The first phase, which correlates with activation of chemotaxis, we call the rapid phase which is activated by both the peptide chemoattractants (fMLP, C5a) and lipid chemoattractants (PAF, LTB_4). This phase involves ligand binding to its receptor which stimulates GTP binding and hence activation of the coupled G protein (Giα2). Pertussis toxin which inactivates certain G proteins is able to block the action of all chemoattractants at this step. The activated G protein causes a phospholipase C-mediated phosphodiesteric cleavage of phosphatidylinositol 4,5-bisphosphate (PIP_2) to form inositol 1,4,5-triphosphate (IP_3) and diacylglycerol (DAG) (Smith et al., 1985, 1986). A phospholipase C is implicated in this step based on analysis of the inositol phosphates produced [i. e. formation of IP_3 coincident with a loss of PIP_2 and later formation of IP and loss of phosphotidylinositol (PI)]. Activation of a phosphoinositide-specific phospholipase C has also been demonstrated for other chemoattractant receptors [C5a, LTB_4, PAF and NAF (IL-8)] (Clancy et al., 1983; Lapetina, 1982; Braquet et al., 1987; Thelen et al., 1988). The IP_3 formed from PIP_2 causes the release of calcium from intracellular stores and the DAG activates protein kinase C. Chelation of intracellular calcium with EGTA attenuates the responses invoked by fMLP implicating a role for calcium in this phase.

The products of the first phase (IP_3 and DAG) may initiate the second sustained phase in the presence of high doses of chemoattractant ($> 10^{-8}$M fMLP or C5a). Activation of this phase correlates with the second function induced by chemoattractants, stimulation of the respiratory burst and exocytosis. Importantly, the peptide chemoattractants (fMLP, C5a) are strong activators of the second phase while lipid chemoattractants (LTB_4, PAF) are poor activators. These discrepences amongst chemoattractants should prove extremely useful in defining the structure-function relationships of their cloned receptors. The second phase is characterized by: (a) an influx of extracellular calcium presumably by activation of a calcium channel via an isomer of IP_3 and subsequently (b) a second, larger and more sustained source of DAG and phosphatidic acid. Protein kinase C involvement is indicated by the fact that fMLP stimulation of this phase results in translocation of protein kinase C activity to the membrane and phorbol esters can mimic certain fMLP generated responses. Fatty acid analysis of DAG produced during the second phase indicates that it arises from hydrolysis of phosphatidylcholine potentially via activation of phospholipase D or a phosphatidylcholine selective-phospholipase C. Involvement of extracellular calcium in initiating this process is supported by the observations that calcium ionophores increase cytosolic calcium levels in leukocytes and stimulate superoxide production, degranulation and DAG production (Truett et al., 1988). Moreover, the second phase is diminished by chelation of extracellular calcium.

While generally protective, the inflammatory process, particularly through the cytotoxic mechanisms of phagocytosis, can lead to severe tissue destruction. Understanding the precise regulation of the locomotive versus cytotoxic potential of leukocytes could lead to more rational designs of anti-inflammatory agents. For example, we have already shown that a hexadecapeptide (mastoporan) can directly activate leukocyte G proteins and biologic activities (Perianin and Snyderman, 1989). Precise definition of receptor-G protein interactions could lead to a more rational design of activators or inhibitors of inflammatory processes.

Association of the formylpeptide receptor with multiple G proteins (i.e. Giα2 and low molecular weight GTP-binding proteins) may be a mechanism by which the receptor governs multiple functions (e.g. chemotaxis and secretion). This possiblility represents a potentially novel and intriguing mechanism of signal transduction. Alternatively, the low molecular weight GTP-binding protein associated with the receptor could mediate receptor trafficking. Cloning and genetic manipulation of chemoattractant receptors will allow us to explore the structure-function relationships of this interesting association with G proteins and should provide new insight into receptor-mediated signal transduction processes.

References

Boulay, F., Tardif, M., Brouchon, L. and Vignais, P. (1990). Bioch. Biophys. Res. Commun. 168: 1103.

Braquet, P. L., Torqui, L., Shen, T. Y. and Vargaftig, B. B. (1987). Pharmacol. Rev. 39: 97.

Clancy, R. M., Dahinden, C. A. and Hugli, T. E. (1983). Proc. Natl. Acad. Sci. USA. 80: 7200.

Hall, A. (1990). Science. 249: 635.

Jesaitis, A. J., Naemura, J. R., Painter, R. G., Sklar, L. A. and Cochrane, C. (1982). Biophys. Biochem. Acta. 719: 556.

Lapetina, E. G. (1982). Trends Pharmacol. Sci. 3: 115.

Polakis, P. G., Evans, T. and Snyderman, R. (1989). Biochem. Biophys. Res. Commun. 161: 276.

Perianin, A. and Snyderman, R. (1989). J. Immunol. 143: 1669.

Smith, C. D., Lane, B. C., Kusaka, I., Verghese, M. W. and Snyderman, R. (1985). J. Biol. Chem. 260: 5875.

Smith, C. D., Cox, C. C. and Snyderman, R. (1986). Science. 232: 97.

Snyderman, R. and Uhing, R. J. (1988). In Inflammation: Basic Principles and Clinical Correlates (Gallin, J. I. Snyderman, R. and Goldstein, I. M., eds.) pp. 303–323.

Snyderman, R., Perianin, A., Evans, T., Polakis, P. and Didsbury, J. R. (1990). "G Proteins and Neutrophil Function". In ADP-Ribosylating Toxins and G Proteins: Insights into Signal Transduction (Moss, J., ed.) American Society for Microbiology, Washington, D.C. pp. 295–323.

Thelen, M., Peveri, P., Kernen, P., Tscharner, V. V., Walz, A. and Baggiolini, M. (1988). FASEB J. 2: 2702.

Truett, A. P., Verghese, M., Dillion, S. B. and Snyderman, R. (1988). Proc. Natl. Acad. Sci. USA 85: 1549.

Regulation of Leukocyte Functions in Inflammation

AAS 35
Progress in Inflammation
Research and Therapy

Conformational Dynamics of the Formyl Peptide Receptor: A Prototype for Studies of Receptor Dynamics and Binding Pocket Structure

L. A. Sklar[1], *S. P. Fay*[1], *H. Mueller*[1], *R. J. Freer*[2], *N. Muthukumaraswamy*[2], *and D. Magde*[3]

[1]Department of Pathology, Cytometry, University of New Mexico School of Medicine, Albuquerque, NM 87131 and National Flow Cytometry Resource, Los Alamos National Laboratory, Los Alamos, NM 87545, USA.
[2]Biomedical Engineering Program, Medical College of Virginia, Virginia Commonwealth University, Richmond, VA 23298-0032, USA.
[3]Department of Chemistry, University of California, San Diego, CA 92093, USA

Summary

We have used spectrofluorometric and flow cytometric techniques to examine the interactions of formyl peptide ligands (L) with their cell surface receptors (R). Kinetic studies suggest that L binds to R at a diffusion limited rate and that R undergoes rapid transitions involving three states (LR, LRG, the ternary complex of L and R with the G protein, and a desensitized receptor "LRX" which forms within seconds) prior to internalization. A spectroscopic analysis of the interaction between L and R show that the binding pocket of R is large enough to contain no more than 6 amino acids and that a fluorescein-labelled pentapeptide is quenched upon binding to R. We hypothesize that histidine 90 (putatively located in the extracellular loop connecting the second and third transmembrane domains) protonates L and quenches the probe. New technology will extend the analysis of structure and dynamics to low affinity peptide receptors of living biological systems. Such technology will have implications in the design of peptidomimetic ligand and drug molecules.

Receptor Dynamics

Cell activation involves a sequence of transient macromolecular assemblies beginning with the binding of stimulatory ligands to cell surface receptors. We have used a combination of spectrofluorometric and flow cytometric approaches to study the interaction of fluorescent derivatives of formyl peptide ligands and their cell surface receptors on human neutrophils (Sklar et al., 1984, 1987, 1989, 1990). This receptor system is likely to be involved in the host defense recognition of peptides released from bacterial membrane proteins.

Neutrophil activation requires an assembly of ternary complex, an interaction among fluorescent peptide ligands (L), receptors (R) and G proteins (G) which we have examined using fluorescence flow cytometry in permeabilized cells. Equilibrium studies showed that LRG binds more tightly by two orders of magnitude than LR. Kinetic studies revealed that this change in affinity was due principally to an increase in the dissociation rate constants for LRG ($1 \times 10^{-3}\,sec^{-1}$) as compared to LR ($1 \times 10^{-1}\,sec^{-1}$). In contrast, the association rate constants for LRG and LR ($2-3 \times 10^{7}\,sec^{-1}M^{-1}$) were statistically indistinguishable and close to the diffusion limit. Kinetic data can be fit with a reaction mechanism for the assembly of the LRG ternary complex in which G is either precoupled to R, or the association of G with LR is fast compared to the association of L with R. The conventional explanation (equation 1) is that to form LRG, ligand first binds to receptor, then receptor finds the G protein and releases the endogenous GDP to form the stable ternary complex. We are evaluating the possibility of pre-coupled RG complexes and the implications of their existence (Fay et al. 1991). In any event, since the receptor is occupied at a diffusion limited rate and ternary complex forms without appreciable delay.

$$L + R \xrightarrow[diffusion]{} LR \xrightarrow[fast]{G} LRG - GDP \xrightarrow[fast]{-GDP} LRG \qquad (1)$$

During cell activation, the ternary complex is activated by the binding of GTP. The rate of dissolution of the ternary complex can be modeled by examining the formation of the rapidly dissociating LR complex from LRG as a function of the concentration of guanine nucleotide. The overall interconversion from LRG to LR occurs at a rate which is proportional to the nucleotide concentration. The results imply that the binding of nucleotide is the rate-limiting step, while the release of activated G protein from LRG occurs rapidly (equation 2). Experiments with GTP indicate that the conversion occurs at a rate of $\sim$10/sec when GTP (500 μM) is near its intracellular level.

$$LRG \xrightarrow[10/\text{sec}]{500\,\mu\text{M}\ GTP} LRG - GTP \xrightarrow[fast]{} LR + G - GTP \qquad (2)$$

The Intact Cell

There are three receptor forms in the intact cell (Sklar et al. 1989). The two forms LRG and LR have been discussed above and the third form is slowly dissociating desensitized receptor ("LRX"). The formation of the desensitized receptor requires energy and receptor occupancy by agonist but does not require G protein, cell activation, or microfilaments (Norgauer et al. 1989). In contrast to the broken cell system, there is a rapid and spontaneous interconversion among the receptor states. The evolution among the receptor states can be probed by adding antagonist at distinct times and then detecting the ligand dissociation. At early times, a rapidly dissociating form similar to LR is followed by a slowly dissociating, desensitized receptor, LRX. After a minute or so of binding only the slow dissociating receptor is detected. Direct measurements of internalization indicate that the slowly dissociating receptor is internalized with a half-time of 3 minutes following a delay of about 30 seconds.

The measured data can be fit with a model based on the direct observation of the behavior of LR and LRG in the permeabilized cell combined with behavior of LRX and internalization in the intact cell (equation 3). The analysis is consistent with these concepts: LRG forms and disappears within a second during cell activation which is too rapid to be detected with the time resolution shown; the intact cell dynamics appear to be dominated by the interconversion between LR and LRX which occurs in several seconds.

$$L + R + G \xrightarrow[diffusion]{} LRG \xrightarrow[>10/\text{sec}]{GTP} LR + G - GTP$$

$$\xrightarrow[\sim 0.1/\text{sec}]{} LRX \xrightarrow[\sim 0.003/\text{sec}]{} LRX\ internal \qquad (3)$$

Receptor dynamics mirror cell responses which are initiated within a few seconds, reach maximal rates of response within tens of seconds, then decay slowly over periods of minutes. When agonist binding is interrupted, it takes a few seconds for the response to be affected, then the response decays. The cell responses decay because the transduction pathway collapses once the active states of the receptor have been lost.

Receptor Binding Pocket Topography

We have studied the topography of interaction of a family of fluorescent formyl peptides containing 4(CHO-met-leu-phe-lys-fluorescein), 5(CHO-met-leu-phe-phe-lys-fluorescein), and 6(CHO-nle-leu-phe-nle-tyr-lys-fluorescein and CHO-met-leu-phe-phe-phe-lys-fluorescein) amino acids with their receptor using spectroscopic methods (Sklar et al. 1990). The fluorescent peptides containing 4 and 5 amino acids were quenched upon binding to the receptor indicating interaction of the chromophore with the receptor. In contrast, the hexapeptides were accessible to antibodies to fluorescein. Taken together, these results suggest that the carboxy terminus of the tetrapeptide or the pentapeptide is protected in the receptor binding pocket while the fluorescein on the carboxy terminus of either hexapeptide is exposed and recognized by the antibody to fluorescein. These results indicate that the binding pocket accommodates at least 5 but not more than 6 amino acids.

In order to understand the structural basis of the quenching interaction in the receptor binding pocket, we have investigated the spectroscopy of the bound fluorescein (Magde and Sklar, unpublished). We examined fluorescence lifetime to determine whether the quenching occurred by a static or dynamic mechanism. In dynamic quenching, the fluorescence lifetime and quantum yield would vary in parallel suggesting that the environment of the fluorescein in the binding pocket was fluctuating on the time frame of the fluorescein lifetime ($\sim$4 nsecs). In the binding pocket however, we detected residual long lifetime rather than intermediate fluorescent lifetime. This result suggests a static mechanism in which the probe coexists in quenched (short lifetime) and unquenched states (long, native lifetime). Two mechanisms can account for coexisting environments: fluorescein can be quenched by a hydrophobic pocket in which case static quenching could require some probe molecules in the pocket and some outside; or, fluorescein can be quenched by protonation in which case coexisting protonated and unprotonated forms would be detected. Fluorescein in a hydrophobic pocket is associated with a red-shifted emission spectrum. In preliminary measurements, no shift of the emission spectrum was detected consistent with the protonation mechanism.

The formyl peptide receptor has been recently cloned and sequenced. The receptor appears to possess seven transmembrane α-helical domains like the β-adrenergic receptor and the photoreceptor rhodopsin. In those receptors the binding pocket is located in a cleft about 1/3 of the way across the membrane bilayer formed by the alpha helical domains. The expected peptide binding region is rich in aromatic amino acids and there is a single histidine (his 90) located ~ 10 Å from the aromatic acid rich binding pocket. His 90 is a good candidate for a protein donor responsible for quenching the fluorescein of the pentapeptide.

Prospects for Generalizing Methods to Low Affinity Peptide Receptors

Fluorescence methodology offers the promise of analyzing ligand-receptor interactions in living systems at the natural abundance of cell surface receptors. The example we discussed, the formyl peptide receptor, can bind agonists with affinities of 10^{10} M^{-1} and there are 50,000 receptors expressed on a fully activated neutrophil.

From a pharmacological perspective it would be desirable to extend the methodology to ligands with affinities as low as 10^6. This range of affinities would encompass most hormone systems, the binding of synthetic peptides and peptidomimetics, and the interactions of new pharmacologic agents. In flow cytometry systems, data acquisition is triggered by the presence of a cell or particle and its accompanying light scatter signal. Flow cytometry is uniquely suited to discriminating the signals of fluorescent ligands associated with cells from ligands in dilute solution surrounding the particles. By incorporating fast mixing capabilities it should be possible to extend these methods to small molecules of affinity 10^6 in which typical association and dissociation rates are predicted to be $>10^7$ $M^{-1}sec^{-1}$ and >10 sec^{-1}. For such low affinity molecules, the equilibration times are governed by the dissociation rates which in general will be in the time frame (half-time) of ~ 100 millisec. Flow detection systems, particularly with new digital data acquisition systems being built at the NFCR, are equipped to function on this time frame. Fast mixing technology has existed for more than 50 years in the physical chemical literature. The next generation of cytometers could function in the time frame of 100's of millisec. A recent demonstration of microsec mixing in cell-sized volumes suggests that it may ultimately become possible to visualize binding mechanisms and receptor structural dynamics associated with binding events in living systems.

References

Fay, S. P., Posner, R. G., Swann, W. N. and Sklar, L. A. (1991). Biochemistry, 30: 5066–5075.

Norgauer, J., Aktories, K. and Sklar, L. A. (1989). J Cell Biology, 109:1133–1140.

Sklar, L. A., Bokoch, G. M., Button, D. and Smolen, J. E. (1987). JBC. 262: 135–139.

Sklar, L. A., Fay, S. P., Seligmann, B. E., Freer, R. J. and Mueller, H. M. (1990). Biochemistry, 29: 313–316.

Sklar, L. A., Finney, D. A., Oades, Z. G., Jesaitis, A. J., Painter, R. G. and Cochrane, C. G. (1984). JBC, 259: 5661–5669.

Sklar, L. A., Mueller, H., Omann, G. M. and Oades, Z. G. (1989). JBC, 264: 8483–8486.

AAS 35
Progress in Inflammation
Research and Therapy

C5a Structural Requirements for Neutrophil Receptor Interaction

*K. W. Mollison, T. A. Fey, R. A. Krause, L. Miller, R. P. Edalji, R. G. Conway, *W. Mandecki, *M. A. Shallcross, M. Kawai, Y. S. Or, B. Lane and G. W. Carter*

Immunoscience Research Area and *Corporate Molecular Biology, Abbott Laboratories, Abbott Park, IL 60064, USA

Summary

A number of C5a modifications were tested to determine effects on receptor binding to polymorphonuclear leukocyte (PMNL) membrane receptors and triggering of PMNL chemokinesis and myeloperoxidase (MPO) release. Site-directed mutagenesis was used to probe relationships of key C-terminal residues, and suggested a role for additional sites, particularly Lys^{19-20}. A synthetic peptide based on C5a 19–30, weakly inhibited C5a binding. Potency of the C-terminal octapeptide, a full agonist, was markedly improved by a single Phe substitution for His^{67}, and a Phe point mutation at this site was shown to enhance activity of the full recombinant protein.

Since the discovery and characterization of C5a as the principal inflammatory mediator derived from complement (reviewed by Hugli, 1984) there has been much therapeutic interest in blocking its effects. To aid design of antagonists, our initial strategy was twofold: (1) determine as much information as possible about which residues of C5a interact with its receptor, using techniques such as site-directed mutagenesis (Mollison et al., 1989) and enzymatic modification (Edalji et al., 1987); and (2) develop structure-activity data from synthetic analogs, commencing with a survey for receptor-binding activity of overlapping peptides (Kawai et al. 1990). For this purpose we focused on the PMNL as a key therapeutic target cell.

Materials and Methods

C5a and analogs: Preparation of rC5a and site-directed mutants was as reported (Mollison et al., 1989). Peptides were made by solid phase synthesis on a 9500 EX or SAM 2 Biosearch synthesizer using Merrifield resin and purified by reversed phase HPLC.

Biologic assays: Cell purification, binding and chemokinesis were as described (Mollison et al., 1989). MPO was measured essentially as reported (Webster and Henson, 1978), except for bringing the cells to 23° after cytochalasin B pretreatment, and using a 1×10^{-6} M rC5a standard.

Results

Figure 1 shows comparative potencies of rC5a mutants for both chemokinesis and MPO release in comparison to their rC5a binding inhibition Ki values. These mutants represent successive residue truncations of the C-terminus from the native 1–74 residues down

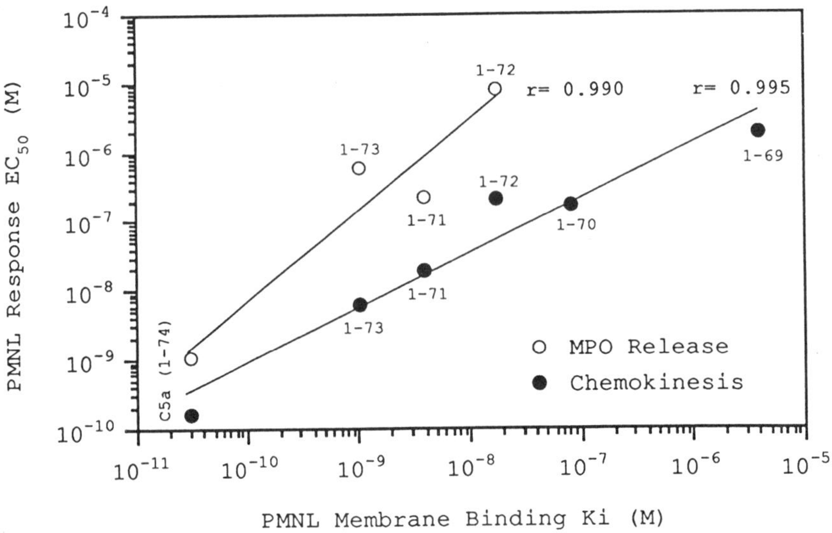

Figure 1. PMNL functional response vs. receptor binding potencies of C5a truncation mutants. Retained residues of the native 1–74 sequence are labeled for each mutant (fitted lines are from analysis by least squares regression)

Table 1. Activities of Modified C5a and Synthetic Peptides

Modification	*PMNL Response: Memb. Binding Ki(nM)*	*Chemokinesis $EC_{50}(nM)$*	*MPO Release $EC_{50}(nM)$*
Native C5a	0.03	0.16	1.1
C5a Asn^{64}, Ile^{65} deleted	0.08	0.23	4.8
C5a Asp^{69} deleted	2.3	3.2	170
C5a 68-Gln-69 insert	0.11	7.3	66
C5a $Lys^{19,20} \rightarrow$ Ser, Ser	19.0	27	2700
19–30 (Cys $\rightarrow$ Ser) peptide	400,000	>1,000,000	N.T.
C5a $His^{67} \rightarrow$ Phe	0.0095	0.02	0.09
His^{67}–74 peptide	300,000	150,000	>1,000,000
Phe^{67}–74 peptide	260	300	37,000

N.T. = not tested

to 1–69. The potencies of the various molecules for inhibiting binding of rC5a to PMNL membranes were highly correlated with their biologic potencies. Although exhibiting differences in sensitivity up to 100-fold, chemokinesis and MPO release activities were concomitantly affected by the various truncations, and both responses showed an inexplicable rank order deviation for 1–71 and 1–72.

Results for other analogs are in Table 1. The binding Kd value for rC5a with PMNL membrane fragments was significantly lower than with intact cells (5×10^{-10} M for the latter). Although chemokinesis was still the most sensitive functional assay, the MPO releasing potencies of rC5a and analogs were typically enhanced 3 to 10-fold by carrying out the procedure at 23° rather than 37° (rC5a $EC_{50} = 8 \times 10^{-9}$ M at 37°).

Discussion

A key aspect in the detection of active, but very low potency peptides and C5a fragments, was the selection of bioassays to maximize sensitivity. Accordingly, PMNL membranes were used routinely for binding competition studies in preference to intact cells and chemokinesis was favored as a functional assay.

Mutants with deletions or insertions among the key residues previously shown to be important for C5a activity, Lys^{68}, Leu^{72} and Arg^{74} (Mollison et al., 1989) exhibited significant potency reductions. This suggests that the native spacing of these key side-chains is critical for maximum potency, although shifting this region as a unit by deleting residues 64 and 65 had little effect on activity.

The ability of mutant rC5a 1–69 not only to bind to the C5a receptor, but also to trigger a functional response supports involvement of areas in addition to the C-terminus in C5a activity. The potency reduction with the double mutation Lys^{19}, Lys^{20} $\rightarrow$ Ser, Ser, and when modified singly (not shown) suggests that these residues are important. Chemical modification (Johnson and Chenoweth, 1985, Hahn, 1987), as well as mutagenesis studies (Mollison et al., 1989) have implicated this region. These results are supported by detection of C5a receptor binding activity by the peptide analog based on residues 19–30, although other peptide analogs based on this region were inactive (Kawai et al., 1989). Its affinity was too weak to permit testing at a high enough concentration to rule out agonist activity.

The Phe-containing C-terminal octapeptide represents a significant advance in maintaining binding potency while reducing molecular size and complexity. The Phe substitution, extremely important in synthetic peptide series (Or et al., 1990), was also found as a point mutation to boost the potency of native rC5a, albeit to a much lesser extent, and presumably interacts with a site on the receptor not normally occupied by the native histidine. Other key functionalities likely resemble features of the native sequence.

Conclusion

Because these studies provide additional evidence that multiple separate regions of C5a interact with the receptor, and that the C-terminus is not required to trigger functional PMNL responses, it was surprising to find that small C-terminal peptide mimics retained full agonist activity. The ease of triggering the C5a receptor by such fragments represents a challenge for design of strict antagonists.

References

Edalji, R. P., Mollison, K. W., Zuiderweg, E. R. P., Fey, T., Krause, R. A., Conway, R. G., Miller, L., Lane, B., Henkin, J., Greer, J. and Carter, G. W. (1987). Truncation of the amino or carboxyl terminus of recombinant C5a reduces receptor binding and biologic activity, Fed. Proc. Exp. Biol. Med. 46: 980.

Hahn, G. S. (1987). U.S. Patent #4,692,511.

Hugli, T. E. (1984). Structure and function of the anaphylatoxins, Springer Semin. Immunopathol. 7: 193–219.

Johnson, R. J. and Chenoweth, D. W. (1985). Structure and function of human C5a anaphylatoxin: selected modification of Tyrosine-23 alters biologic activity but not antigenicity, J. Biol. Chem. 260: 10339–10345.

Kawai, M., Quincy, D. A., Lane, B., Mollison, K. W., Luly, J. R., and Carter, G. W. (1990). Identification of a receptor binding region of the human anaphylatoxin C5a, 199th ACS National Meeting, April 22–27, Boston, MA, Div. Med. Chem., 87.

Mollison, K. W., Mandecki, W., Zuiderweg, E. R. P., Fayer, L., Fey, T., Krause, R. A., Conway, R. G., Miller, L., Edalji, R. P., Shallcross, M. A., Lane, B., Fox, J. L., Greer, J. and Carter, G. W. (1989). Identification of receptor binding residues in the inflammatory complement protein C5a by site-directed mutagenesis, PNAS, USA 86: 292–296.

Or, Y. S., Clark, R. F., Kawai, M., Mollison, K. W., Lane, B., Luly, J. and Carter, G. W. (1990). Improvements in the minimum binding sequence of C5a, 200th ACS National Meeting, Aug. 26–31, Washington, D.C., Div. Med. Chem., 176.

Webster, R. O. and Henson, P. M. (1978). Rapid measurement of neutrophil exocytosis, Inflammation 3: 129–135.

AAS 35
Progress in Inflammation
Research and Therapy

Adhesion-Promoting Receptors on Phagocytes

S. D. Wright

Laboratory of Cellular Physiology and Immunology, The Rockefeller University, 1230 York Avenue, New York, NY 10021, USA

Summary

In order for leukocytes to migrate to sites of inflammation they must first adhere to the vascular endothelium. This initial adhesion, however, must be rapidly broken to allow diapedesis. Recent studies have shown that the CD18 family of leukocyte integrins plays a pivotal role in the transient adhesions needed for diapedesis. The means by which CD18 molecules mediate transient adhesion and the respective roles of CD18 molecules and other adhesion molecules in inflammation are discussed.

The CD18 family of leukocyte integrins: Leukocytes express a family of three cell-surface glycoproteins, CD11a/CD18 (LFA-1), CD11b/CD18 (CR3), and CD11c/CD18 (p150,95), that perform a broad range of adhesive functions (Wright & Detmers, 1988). Each of the three molecules is composed of one alpha chain (~ 180 kDa) and one beta chain (95 kDa). Both chains are transmembrane proteins with a small cytoplasmic portion, a single membrane-spanning domain, and a large exoplasmic domain. The beta chain (CD18) is identical for all three members, while the alpha chains are homologous but distinct proteins.

LFA-1 is expressed on all leukocytes and mediates the adhesion of cytotoxic T cells to targets and the interaction of PMN with endothelium. It binds to the broadly distributed ligand, ICAM-1 as well as to additional but less well characterized proteins.

CR3 is restricted to phagocytes and mediates attachment of these cells to endothelium as well as to surfaces coated with a variety of ligands. CR3 was first recognized for its ability to bind particles coated with the complement fragment C3bi and serves as an opsonic receptor. The name CR3 (complement receptor type 3) reflects this capacity. In addition, CR3 recognizes surfaces coated with fibrinogen, and the microbial proteins gp63 of *Leishmania* and filamentous hemagluttinin of *Bordetella pertussis*. The latter recognition specificities are likely to enable these microbes to establish a parasitic infection of macrophages.

P150,95 is expressed on phagocytes and murine dendritic cells, but its precise function is not known.

The CD18 molecules are members of a larger, broadly distributed family of proteins that promote cell adhesion. This class of molecules, termed "integrins," includes the fibronectin receptor (and other members of the VLA antigen series), the vitronectin receptor, gp IIb/IIIa of platelets, and several others. All integrins show strong structural homology and all share the capacity to mediate adhesive interactions. Leukocytes express integrins in addition to CD18, but since CD18 molecules are present only on leukocytes, they are often referred to as "the leukocyte integrins."

CD18 molecules are necessary for movement of PMN to sites of inflammation: The role of CD18 molecules in immune responses is highlighted by observations on patients who have a congenital deficiency in CD18 termed Leukocyte Adhesion Deficiency (LAD) (Todd & Freyer, 1988). Leukocytes from affected individuals are deficient in a number of adhesion functions assayed in vitro. The principal consequence of this deficiency is a strong predisposition to infection. Of particular note is that polymorphonuclear leukocytes (PMN) fail to move to sites of inflammation and pus does not form. These observations suggest that the functioning of CD18 molecules is vital for the movement of PMN out of the vasculature.

The symptoms of LAD may be reproduced in animals by injection of an antibody against CD18. Animals treated in this way fail to mobilize PMN to inflammatory sites in the skin, brain, heart, and peritoneal cavity (Arfors et al., 1987; Simpson et al., 1988; Tuomanen et al., 1989). Because of the very striking nature of the inhibition caused by anti-CD18 antibodies, they have been proposed as potential anti-inflammatory agents.

Adhesion mediated by CD18 molecules is transient: PMN must bind to endothelium to emmigrate from the vasculature, but it is clear this adhesive capacity must be held in abeyance for the cells to circulate. Further, the adhesion to endothelium must be broken in order for cells to move away from the endothelium and into tissues. The CD18 molecules are uniquely suited to mediate the transient, regulated adhesion required by these cells. Unstimulated PMN express CD18 molecules that are incapable of binding any of their known ligands (C3bi, fibrinogen, ICAM-1, or other ligands on endothelium) (Wright & Meyer, 1986; Lo et al., 1989). Within less than a minute after being exposed to a chemotactic factor such as C5a, TNF, fMLP, or PMA, the CD18 molecules become capable of mediating adhesion. The "activation" of receptors is transient, and binding activity returns to baseline in 15–40 minutes depending on the agonist. CD18 molecules may undergo successive cycles of activation and deactivation, and we have proposed that cycles of CD18-mediated adhesion (at the leading front of a cell) and release (at the uropod) function in locomotion.

Recent studies have described molecules on endothelium (GMP-140, ELAM-1, and PAF) that may serve in recruitment of PMN to sites of inflammation. The precise contribution of these molecules, however, has been uncertain since migration of PMN is *entirely* dependent on CD18 molecules, and none of the endothelial cell molecules above serve as ligands for CD18. Recent studies from our laboratory suggest a mechanism by which endothelial adhesins such as ELAM-1 and the CD18 molecules of PMN can function together to promote diapedesis (Lo et al., 1991). We have found that interaction of PMN with ELAM-1 causes strong activation of CD18 molecules. Thus, an initial interaction of PMN with ELAM-1 may recruit adhesive interactions mediated by CD18, which can then serve in the cycles of adhesion and release necessary for diapedesis. Two types of adhesion molecules may thus function in series, not parallel, to target PMN to sites of inflammation.

Acknowledgements

I wish to thank Dr. Patricia A. Detmers for critical reading of the manuscript. This work was supported by USPHS grants AI-22003 and AI-24775. The author is an Established Investigator of the American Heart Association.

References

Arfors, K.-E., Lundberg, C., Lindblom, L., Lundberg, K., Beatty, P. G. and Harlan, J. M. (1987). A monoclonal antibody to the membrane glycoprotein complex CD18 inhibits polymorphonuclear leukocyte accumulation and plasma leakage in vivo. Blood 69: 338–340.

Lo, S. K., Detmers, P. A., Levin, S. M. and Wright, S. D. (1989). Transient adhesion of neutrophils to endothelium. J. Exp. Med. 169: 1779–1793.

Lo, S. K., Lee, S., Ramos, R., Lobb, R. Rosa, M., Chi-Rosso, G., and Wright, S. D. (1991). Endothelial-Leukocyte adhesion molecule 1 stimulates the adhesive activity of leukocyte integrin CR3 (CD11b/CD18, Mac-1, $\alpha_m\beta_2$) on human neutrophils, J. Exp. Med. 173: 1493–1500.

Simpson, P. J., Todd, R. F., III, Fantone, J. C., Mickelson, J. K., Griffin, J. D. and Luccesi, B. R. (1988). Reduction of experimental canine myocardial reperfusion injury by a monoclonal antibody (Anti-Mo1, Anti-CD11b) that inhibits leukocyte adhesion. J. Clin. Invest. 81: 624–629.

Todd, R. F., III and Freyer, D. R. (1988). The CD11/CD18 leukocyte glycoprotein deficiency. Hem./Onc. Clin. N. Amer. 2: 13–31.

Tuomanen, E. I., Saukkonen, K., Sande, S., Cioffe, C. and Wright, S. D. (1989). Reduction of inflammation, tissue damage, and mortality in bacterial meningitis in rabbits treated with monoclonal antibodies against adhesion-promoting receptors of leukocytes. J. Exp. Med. 170: 959–968.

Wright, D. S. and Detmers, P. A. (1988). Adhesion-promoting receptors on phagocytes. J. Cell. Sci. Suppl. 9: 99–120.

Wright, S. D. and Meyer, B. C. (1986). Phorbol esters cause sequential activation and deactivation of complement receptors on polymorphonuclear leukocytes. J. Immunol. 136: 1759–1764.

Cytokines

AAS 35
Progress in Inflammation
Research and Therapy

Cytokine Modulation of Bacterial Cell Wall-Induced Arthritis

S. M. Wahl, J. B. Allen and M. E. Brandes

Cellular Immunology Section, National Institute of Dental Research, National Institutes of Health, Bethesda, MD 20892, USA

Summary

Bacterial cell wall-induced arthritis in experimental animals is dependent on mononuclear cell infiltration and accumulation. These mononuclear cells secrete cytokines which promote synovial hyperplasia and erosive destruction of bone and cartilage. Whereas local administration of cytokines may exacerbate these events, systemic administration of TGF-β or γIFN effectively suppresses both the acute and chronic phases of the disease.

Initiation of synovitis in susceptible rats is dependent upon dissemination of injected bacterial cell walls to the synovium (Cromartie et al., 1977). Once localized in the synovium, the bacterial cell walls from group A streptococcus (SCW) activate complement (Schwab et al., 1982) and trigger recruitment of leukocytes from the circulation into the synovial tissues. The erythema and swelling characteristic of the acute response transiently subside and mononuclear cells migrate into the synovial tissue as the chronic, destructive phase of the disease begins. The mechanism responsible for the acute and chronic aspects of the lesion have been shown to be distinct and independently susceptible to regulation by pharmacologic agents and biological response modifiers (Allen et al., 1985).

To further explore the mechanisms of synovial inflammation for the purpose of identifying site specific inhibitors which may be relevant to suppressing synovial inflammatory events in rheumatoid disease, we have recently analyzed the effects of local and systemic administration of certain cytokines on the course of the disease. In particular, whereas TGF-β injected locally promoted synovial inflammation, intraperitoneal injection significantly suppressed arthritis (Allen et al., 1990a; Brandes et al., 1991). Similarly, γIFN was an effective therapeutic agent when administered systemically, but its local administration elicited pro-inflammatory effects (Allen et al., 1991b; Wahl, S. et al., 1991).

Materials and Methods

Induction and Monitoring of Arthritis: Specific pathogen-free female Lewis rats (Harlan Sprague Dawley, Indianapolis, IN) ($\sim$100 gm) were injected intraperitoneally (i.p.) with an aqueous bacterial cell wall preparation isolated from Group A streptococci. The development of clinical arthritis was monitored daily and quantitated as an articular index (AI) based on the degree of erythema, swelling and deformity (Allen et al., 1991b). Each extremity was graded on a scale of 0–4.

Administration of cytokines: Purified recombinant rodent γIFN (Amgen, Thousand Oaks, CA) was injected i.p. at 10^5 units/animal (Allen et al., 1991b) or intra-articularly (i.a.) at 10^4 units/25 μl. To test the effects of TGF-β on the development of arthritis, TGF-β was injected i.p. daily at 0.1–5.0 μg/2 ml/animal for intervals specified for each experiment or administered i.a. from 0.1–1 μg/50 μl. The TGFβ stock was diluted in a carrier solution of rat serum albumin in PBS (1 mg/ml) immediately prior to i.p. administration. Control animals received an equal volume of PBS or the relevant carrier.

Histopathology: Synovial specimens were dissected, fixed in 2% glutaraldehyde and 2% formaldehyde and postfixed with 1% OsO_4. After embedding in Spurr epoxy resin, the tissues were sectioned and stained with toluidine blue for examination by light microscopy.

Results

Effect of TGF-β on Acute and Chronic Arthritis: Joints exhibiting inflammation due to SCW deposition responded to the i.a. injection of TGF-β with a pronounced exacerbation of the arthritic condition (Table 1). Although the maximum inflammation typically observed during SCW-induced arthritis is scored as a 4, local administration of a single injection of 250 ng TGF-β augmented the inflammation beyond these levels. After cessation of TGF-β, no amelioration of inflammation or augmentation of tissue healing was evident in the treated animals.

Table I. Effect of Local and Systemic Administration of TGF-β on SCW Arthritis

*Treatment**	*Articular Index* *Acute*	*Chronic*
Vehicle	4	4
TGF-β (250 ng, i.a.)	>4	>4
TGF-β (1.0 μg, i.p.)	0.5	1

*SCW-injected animals received TGF-β or the appropriate vehicle either i.a. in a single 250 ng injection or i.p. at 1 μg/2 ml/day. Articular indices for individual joints were determined on day 3–5 (acute) and day 14–16 (chronic).

In contrast to local injection of TGF-β, systemic administration of the polypeptide was found to markedly inhibit the development of polyarthritis in the SCW-injected rats. When i.p. TGF-β injections were begun one day prior to the SCW and continued on a daily basis, joint swelling and deformity during the acute phase were suppressed (Table I). Moreover, the chronic phase of the disease was virtually eliminated (Table I, Brandes et al., 1991). Control animals receiving only TGF-β displayed no discernable effects. Histological examination of the tissue revealed that TGF-β suppressed the infiltration of inflammatory cells, pannus formation and joint erosion. TGF-β also suppressed the evolution of arthritis even when administration was begun after the acute phase of the disease (day 10). Immunological function in animals treated with TGF-β appeared intact; however, TGF-β inhibited the leukocytosis associated with the chronic phase of arthritis. These observations suggested that systemic administration of TGF-β suppresses arthritis by reducing the reservoir of circulating leukocytes available for recruitment into the joints. In addition, systemic TGF-β may act to eliminate the TGF-β chemotaxis gradient at the site of inflammation.

Effect of Recombinant γIFN on Acute and Chronic Arthritis: γIFN has been shown to have both pro- and anti-inflammatory effects (Nathan & Yoshida, 1988). Local injection of γIFN into an inflamed synovium was shown to cause an augmentation of the inflammatory response. Injection of 10^4 units γIFN/joint at either the acute or chronic stage resulted in an increase in the AI from 3.5 to >4, the maximum achievable AI (Table II). This increased AI was reflected by increased leukocyte accumulation and activation within the synovium. In contrast, recent studies evaluating the therapeutic efficacy of systemic γIFN on the development of SCW-induced erosive polyarthritis demonstrated a reduction in the AI (Table II) by 80% compared to the SCW-injected control animals during the acute response. This γIFN-mediated suppression of synovial inflammation was maintained into the chronic phase of the arthritis, and furthermore, suppressed the normally persistent, erosive phase of the lesions (Allen et al., 1991b).

Histologically, on days 3–5, normally the peak of the acute response to SCW, those animals receiving γIFN therapy exhibited a marked reduction in the number of infiltrating inflammatory neutrophils and monocytes. Moreover, during the chronic, mononuclear cell-dependent phase of the arthritis, the level of mononuclear phagocytes in the synovial tissues remained very low in the γIFN-treated as compared to the untreated arthritic animals. This reduction in cellular infiltrate was consistent with the diminished clinical and histopathologic parameters and suggested that the γIFN was influencing recruitment of circulating leukocytes into the local inflammatory site (Wahl et al., 1991).

Table II. Effect of Local and Systemic Administration of γIFN on SCW Arthritis

*Treatment**	*Articular Index*	
	Acute	*Chronic*
Vehicle	3.5	4
γIFN (10^4 units i.a.)	>4	>4
γIFN (10^5 units i.p.)	2	1

*SCW-injected animals received γIFN or the appropriate vehicle either i.a. in a single dose of 10^4 units or i.p. at 10^5 units/day. Articular indices for individual joints were determined on day 3–5 (acute) and day 14–16 (chronic).

Discussion

The induction of polyarthritis by bacterial cell products (SCW) provides an important experimental model for dissecting acute and chronic aspects of the immune response leading to connective tissue degradation. Importantly, it also provides a reproducible system to evaluate certain therapeutic modalities for their effects on both acute inflammatory events and on the chronic phases of an immune response which occur by distinct cellular and molecular mechanisms. In the current studies, we have shown that two immunomodulatory cytokines, γIFN and TGF-β, with distinct mechanisms of action can profoundly influence the course of bacterial cell wall induced erosive polyarthritis. Moreover, it is clear that the route of administration of these biological response modifiers determines their impact on the inflammatory events. In this regard, γIFN administered directly into the articular space increased the synovial inflammatory response, whereas systemic injection of the cytokine resulted in an effective therapeutic reduction in the arthritis.

Mechanistically, several distinct, but related mechanisms may mediate the γIFN suppression of arthritis. For example, γIFN suppress inflammatory cell recruitment by its ability to suppress complement activation (Lotz & Zuraw, 1987; Hamilton et al., 1987), prostaglandin synthesis (Wahl, L. et al., 1990) and monocyte chemotaxis (Wahl, S. et al., 1990). Moreover, γIFN inhibits synovial cell hyperplasia (Allen et al., 1990b) minimizing pannus formation and blocks collagenase synthesis (Wahl, L. et al., 1990). In sum, γIFN can suppress several aspects of inflammation relevant to the acute and chronic responses to antigen, and in so doing, markedly inhibits arthritis in the SCW model. These results are consistent with its therapeutic effects in recent rheumatoid arthritis clinical trials (Lemmel et al., 1987; Cannon et al., 1988).

Although TGF-β clearly has distinct mechanisms of action from γIFN, TGF-β also dramatically antagonized the SCW-induced arthritis when administered systemically corresponding to its numerous immunosuppressive activities (Wahl et al., 1988, 1989). The evidence obtained thus far towards delineating its anti-arthritic mechanisms suggest that active TGF-β in the circulation suppresses SCW-induced leukocytosis, and eliminates the chemotactic concentration gradient normally emanating from the inflamed synovium. Thus, these two cytokines, by distinct mechanisms of action and without apparent toxicity, appear to be influential in ameliorating inflammatory and immunological sequelae of SCW deposition in the synovium. As the mechanisms of action of these two disparate cytokines continue to be delineated, additional insight into therapeutic modalities appropriate for arthropathies and other chronic inflammatory lesions may emerge.

References

Allen, J. B., Malone, D. G., Wahl, S. M., Calandra, G. B., and Wilder, R. L. (1985). J. Clin Invest 76: 1042–1056.

Allen, J. B., Manthey, C. L., Hand, A. R., Ohura, K., Ellingsworth, L., and Wahl, S. M. (1990a). J. Exp. Med. 171: 231–247.

Allen, J. B., Bansal, G., Feldman, G. M., Hand, A. O., Wahl, L. M., and Wahl, S. M. (1991). Cytokine 3: 98–106.

Brandes, M. E., Allen, J. B., Ogawa, Y., and Wahl, S. M. (1991). J. Clin. Invest. 87: 1108–1113.

Cannon, G. W., Pincus, S. H., Emkey, R. D., Denes, A., Cohen, S. A., Wolfe, A., Saway, P. A., Jaffer, A. M., Wearer, A. L., Cogen, L., and Schindler, J. D. (1988). Arthritis Rheum. 32: 964–973.

Cromartie, W. J., Craddock, J. G., Schwab, J. H., Anderle, S. K., and Yang, C. H. (1977). J. Exp. Med. 146: 1585–1602.

Hamilton, A. O., Jones, L., Morrison, L., and Whaley, K. (1987). Biochem. J. 242: 809–815.

Lemmel, E. M., Brackertz, D., Franke, M., Gaus, W., Hartl, P. W., Machalke, K., Mielke, K., Obert, H. J., Peter, H. H., Sieper, J., Sprekeler, R., and Stierle, H. (1987). Rheumatol. Int. 8: 87–93.

Lotz, M., and Zuraw, B. L. (1987). J. Immunol. 139: 3382–3387.

Nathan, C. F., and Yoshida, R. (1988). In Inflammation: Basic Principles and Clinical Correlates. J. I. Gallin, I. M. Goldstein, R. Snyderman, eds. Raven Press, New York, p. 229–51.

Schwab, J. H., Allen, J. B., Anderle, S. K., Dalldorf, F., Eisenberg, R., and Cromartie, W. J. (1982). Immunology 46: 83–89.

Wahl, L. M., Corcoran, M. L., Mergenhagen, S. E., and Finbloom, D. S. (1990). J. Immunol. 144: 3518–3522.

Wahl, S. M., Hunt, D. A., Wong, H. L., Dougherty, S., McCartney-Francis, N., Wahl, L. M., Ellingsworth, L., Schmidt, J. A., Hall, G., Roberts, A. B., and Sporn, M. B. (1988). J. Immunol. 140: 3026–3032.

Wahl, S. M., McCartney-Francis, N., and Mergenhagen, S. E. (1989). Immunology Today 10: 258–261.

Wahl, S. M., Allen, J. B., Ohura, K., Chenoweth, D. E., and Hand, A. R. (1991). J. Immunol. 146: 95–100.

AAS 35
Progress in Inflammation
and Research and Therapy

Interleukin 1 Signal Transduction

J. Saklatvala and F. Guesdon

Cytokine Biochemistry Department, Strangeways Research Laboratory, Worts Causeway, Cambridge CB1 4RN, UK

Summary

Interleukin 1 signals through an 80kDa receptor to change protein kinase activity in fibroblasts. Two increases in protein phosphorylation have been identified: the EGF receptor and the small heat shock protein (hsp 27). Both involve serine and are similarly transient (maximal 5–15 minutes). The kinase activity differs from PKA or C. Hsp 27 can be used for its assay in extracts of stimulated cells.

Interleukin 1 controls the behaviour of a variety of cell types in inflammatory and immune responses. Its multiple physiological actions are now well recognised.

The cytokine acts by inducing synthesis of specific proteins, the nature of which depends on the type of responding cell. How are such cell-specific and cytokine-specific responses determined at a biochemical level? The molecular mechanisms by which IL1 activates cells are not clear. Virtually all known signalling systems have been implicated, and the area is highly controversial.

Interleukin 1 Receptors

There are two distinct plasma membrane recptors for IL1. Early experiments revealed an 80kDa receptor protein on T cell lines and various types of fibroblast (Dower *et al.*, 1985; Bird and Saklatvala, 1986). This protein when purified in soluble form bound IL1 with the same affinity as the receptor in the cell membrane (Bird *et al.*, 1988). The protein has been cloned and is a member of the immunoglobulin superfamily (Sims *et al.*, 1988, 1989). It has a single transmembrane region and its cytoplasmic portion has no recognisably regulatable fuction: the cloned protein transmits an IL1 signal. Its extracellular part is heavily glycosylated, and binds IL1α or β with similar affinity.

Early cross-linking experiments showed that B lymphocytes and B cell lines had a smaller receptor (Matsushima *et al.*, 1986). Recent work has shown that this 67kDa protein is a second receptor, distinct from the first (Bomsztyk *et al.*, 1989; Chizzonite *et al.*, 1989). Its signalling fuction has yet to be established. As far as is known there is no relationship between the IL1 receptors and those for TNF (see article by Dr Wallach) although the two cytokines have very similar effects.

IL1 Changes Gene Expression

IL1 increases expression of specific genes in target cells. Many of these changes are also induced by TNF and are mimicked by the tumour promoter phorbol myristate acetate (PMA). PMA, IL1 and TNF all induce or activate similar transcription factors which bind to specific sites in the 5′ regulatory regions of responsive genes. They induce c-jun, which binds to AP1 sites. AP1-regulated genes include stromelysin, collagenase and IL2 (Muegge and Durrum, 1990). All three also activate nuclear factor kappa B (NFkB) in cells (Osborn *et al.* 1989). Genes regulated by this transcription factor include kappa immunoglobin chains and the IL2 receptor a chain (Muegge and Durrum, 1990).

Protein phosphorylation is thought to underly activation of these systems: in the case of NFkB there is phosphorylation of an inhibitory protein (IkB) which releases active NFkB (Ghosh and Baltimore, 1990). The mechanism of induction of AP1 binding proteins is not known. PMA activates protein kinase C, and because of the biological similarities between PMA, IL1 and TNF it has always seemed likely that the cytokines work by activating that kinase or a functionally similar enzyme.

IL1 Activates a Serine Kinase

IL1 rapidly increases a protein kinase activity in fibroblasts: two changes in protein phosphorylation, both involving serine, have been identified.

We found accidentally that IL1 rapidly lowered the affinity of the epidermal growth factor (EGF) receptor on fibroblasts for its ligand (Bird and Saklatvala, 1988). The effect of IL1 was associated with an increase in phosphorylation (mainly of serine) of the EGF receptor (Bird and Saklatvala, 1989 and 1990). Tumour necrosis factor (TNF) had the same effect. Such transmodulation can also be caused by treating cells with PMA.

The cytokine-induced phosphorylation of the EGF receptor differed from that due to PMA in that:

(i) it did not inhibit the tyrosine kinase activity of the receptor which is induced by binding EGF.

(ii) it occurred in cells which had been depleted of protein kinase C.

(iii) it was not inhibited by staurosporine, a potent inhibitor of protein kinase C.

(iv) phosphopeptide maps of the EGF receptor from cytokine-stimulated or PMA-stimulated cells showed marked differences.

These results suggested that IL1 and TNF stimulated a kinase(s) other than protein kinase C. Transmodulation desensitizes the cell to the growth factor, but the significance of this for cytokine action is not known. Nevertheless, the phosphorylation state of the EGF receptor provided us with an indicator of changes in kinase activity inside the stimulated cells.

The second increase in protein phosphorylation which we identified in IL1-stimulated fibroblasts involved the small heat shock protein, hsp 27. Fig. 1 shows the phosphoproteins of MRC5 fibroblasts. The cells had been metabolically labelled with [^{32}P]-orthophosphate then stimulated by IL1 or TNF. The cytokines increased phosphorylation of three phosphoproteins marked (a) – (c). These have been shown to be forms of hsp 27 (Kaur *et al*, 1989).

Hsp 27 is a constitutive cytosolic protein homologous to a crystallin but its function is unclear (Arrigo *et al.*, 1988). Its synthesis is induced strongly by exposing cells to temperatures 4–5 °C above normal and it may protect against thermal injury (Landry *et al.*, 1989).

In resting MRC5 fibroblasts 10–15% of the protein is phosphorylated; upon stimulation of the cells with IL1 this increases to about 85%. De-phosphorylation occurs slowly over the subsequent hour

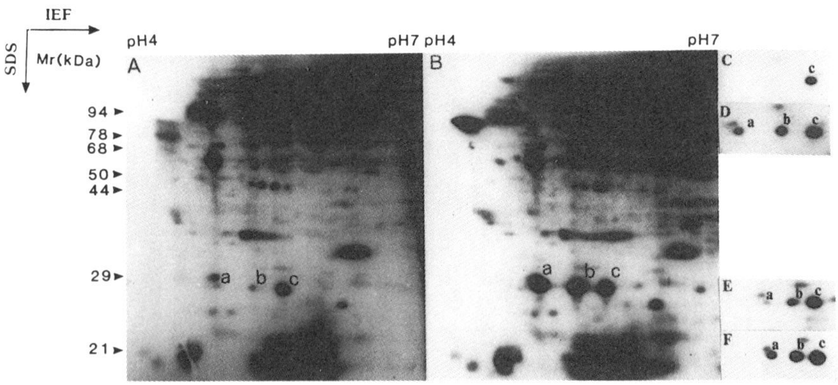

Figure 1. MRC5 fibroblasts labelled to equilibrium (8 h) with [^{32}P] orthophosphate were stimulated for 10 min, washed and scraped into 3% TCA. Pellets were dissolved in 8 M urea and 1% NP40 and subjected to 2 D electrophoresis. Autoradiographs show the three phosphorylated forms of hsp 27 marked (a) – (c). For details of the procedures see Kaur *et al.* (1988 and 1989). (A,C.E) controls; (B) IL1α; (D) TNF; (F) IL1β.

or two. Phosphoamino acid analysis shows that all three forms contain only phosphoserine (Kaur *et al.*, 1989).

IL1 induces this phosphorylation in cells other than fibroblasts: it is seen in chondrocytes, vascular endothelial cells and the hepatoma line, HepG2. Additionally, TNF is able to induce it in U937 cells.

As in the case of the EGF receptor the kinase responsible for the phosphorylation of hsp 27 appears to be distinct from protein kinase C. PMA stimulates phosphorylation of hsp 27 but its effect is less marked than IL1. When cells are depleted of kinase C by prolonged treatment with PMA the response to IL1 is unaffected (Kaur and Saklatvala, unpublished observations).

The similarity in time course of the phosphorylation of hsp 27 and the EGF receptor, and the fact that both involve serine, suggests they might be due to the same kinase. Whether the kinase is involved in activating or inducing the transcription factors described earlier remains to be seen. It is highly unlikely that IL1 works by activating a single kinase!

Hsp 27, which is a small cytosolic protein, is potentially a convenient substrate for characterizing and isolating and IL1- or

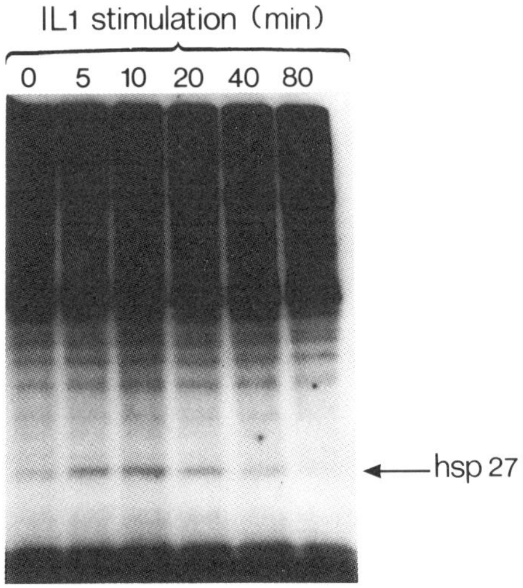

Figure 2. MRC5 fibroblasts were taken up in 25 mM Tris, 0.1% NP40, 0.1 mM EDTA, 0.1 mM EGTA, 1 mM PMSF, pH 7.5, and microfuged. 4 vol. of supernatant was mixed with one of extract of cells stimulated by IL1 for the indicated times. [^{32}P] gamma ATP (2 micromolar final) and $MgCl_2$ (8 mM final) were added and mixtures incubated for 30 min at 37 °C. Reaction was stopped by adding SDS (0.1% final) and heating at 100 °C for 3 min. Samples were run on SDS-PAGE; dried gels were autoradiographed.

TNF-inducible serine kinase. We carried out experiments to detect such a kinase. One volume of extract of stimulated cells was mixed with four volumes of extracts of unstimulated cells and [^{32}P]ATP.

Fig. 2 shows that hsp 27-phosphorylating activity was detected in the stimulated extracts. It was transient, being maximal between 5 and 20 minutes after stimulation. We are currently purifying hsp 27 to use as a substrate for a cytokine-induced kinase assay.

IL1, Second Messengers and G Proteins

How are IL1-responsive kinases regulated? In agreement with many laboratories we have failed to find increases in either cAMP or diacylglycerol in cells responding to IL1. This is consistent with our view that the cytokine-activated kinase is neither A nor C.

The earliest event which we have detected in response to IL1 is activation of a GTP-binding protein(s) in a strain (NOB1) of the murine thymoma line EL4 (O'Neill *et al.*, 1990). The significance of this for the activation of protein kinase or other signalling mechanisms is unknown.

Acknowledgements

We are grateful to the Arthritis Council and Medical Research Council, both of the UK, for financial support.

References

Arrigo, A. P., Suchan. J. and Welch, W. J. (1988). Mol. Cell Biol. 8: 5059–5071.
Bird, T. A. and Saklatvala, J. (1986). Nature 324: 263–265.
Bird, T. A. and Saklatvala, J. (1988). J. Immunol. 142: 126–133.
Bird, T. A. and Saklatvala, J. (1990). J. Biol. Chem. 265: 235–240.
Bird, T. A., Gearing, A. J. H. and Saklatvala, J. (1988). J. Biol. Chem. 263: 12063–12069.
Bomsztyk, K., Sims, J. E., Stanton, T. H., Slack, J., McMahon, C. J., Valentine, M. A. and Dower, S. K. (1989). Proc. Natl. Acad. Sci, U.S.A. 86: 8033–8038.
Chizzonite, R., Truitt, T., Kilian, P. L., Stern, A. S., Nunes, P., Parker, K., Kaffka, K. L., Chua, A. O., Lugg, D. K. and Gubler, U. (1989). Proc. Natl. Acad. Sci, U.S.A. 86: 8029–8033.
Dower, S. L., Kronheim, S. R., March, C. J., Conlon, P. J., Hopp, T. P., Gillis, S. and Urdal, D. (1985). J. Exp. Med. 162: 505–515.
Ghosh, S. and Baltimore, D. (1990). Nature 344: 678–682.
Landry, J., Chrétien, P., Lambert, H., Hickey, E. and Weber, L. A. (1989). J. Cell Biol. 109: 7–15.
Kaur, P. and Saklatvala, J. (1988). FEBS Lett. 241: 6–10.
Kaur, P., Welch, W. J. and Saklatvala (1989). FEBS Lett. 258: 269–273.
Matsushima, K., Akahoshi, T., Yamada, M., Furutani, Y. and Oppenheim, J. J. (1986). J. Immunol. 136: 4496–4501.
Muegge, K. and Durum, S. (1990). Cytokine 2: 1–18.
O'Neill, L. A. J., Bird, T. A., Gearing, A. J. H. and Saklatvala, J. (1990). J. Biol. Chem. 265: 3146–3152.
Osborn, L., Kunkel, S. and Nabel, G. J. (1989). Proc. Natl. Acad. Sci, U.S.A. 86: 2336–2340.
Sims, J. E., March, C. J., Cosman, D., Widmer, M. B., MacDonald, H. R., McMahon, C. J., Grubin, C. E., Wignall, J. M., Jackson, J. L., Call, S. M., Friend, D., Alpert, A. R., Gillis, S., Urdal, D. L. and Dower, S. K. (1988). Science, 241: 585–589.
Sims, J. E., Acres, R. B., Grubin, C. E., McMahon, C. J., Wignall, J. M., March, C. J. and Dower, S. K. (1989). Proc. Natl. Acad. Sci, U.S.A. 86: 8946–8950.

AAS 35
Progress in Inflammation
Research and Therapy

IL-1ra: Properties and Uses of an Interleukin-1 Receptor Antagonist

R. C. Thompson, D. J. Dripps, and S. P. Eisenberg

Synergen, Inc., 1885 33rd Street, Boulder, CO 80301, USA

Interleukin-1α and *β* are thought to be mediators of a range of inflammatory diseases either because levels of these cytokines increase in the course of the disease or because exogenous IL-1 can induce some aspects of the disease. To test this hypothesis we should examine whether the course of a disease can be interrupted by specific inhibitors of interleukin 1 action. Several agents are now being developed which have this property including an antibody to the mouse type I IL-1 receptor (Chizzonite et al., 1989), a soluble form of the Type I IL-1 receptor (Sims et al., 1988), and an *interleukin-1 receptor antagonist* (IL-1ra) (Hannum et al., 1990; Eisenberg et al., 1990). In this article we attempt to summarise what is known about the receptor antagonist and describe how it acts as a specific inhibitor of IL-1 action *in vitro* and *in vivo*. We then describe the results of experiments using IL-1ra that confirm the role of IL-1 in animal models of *inflammatory bowel disease* and *septic shock*.

The presence of the protein now known as IL-1ra was first noted by J-M Dayer in the urine from monoblastic leukemia patients (Balavoine et al., 1984; 1986) and by Bill Arend in the medium conditioned by monocytes grown on immune complexes (Arend et al., 1985). Following his initial observations Dayer partially purified the material and showed that it acted on the target cell rather than on the IL-1 itself and postulated that it acted as a *receptor antagonist* (Seckinger et al., 1987). The Synergen group became associated with this protein through our search for agents which would prevent cartilage destruction and we formed a collaboration with Bill Arend with the goal of purifying and determining the structure of the IL-1 inhibitor. To accomplish this Chuck Hannum purified several micrograms of active protein from monocyte conditioned medium and obtained sufficient sequence for us to clone the cDNA from a human monocyte library (Hannum et al., 1990; Eisenberg et al., 1990). Subsequent to this work Carter et al., (1990) isolated an IL-1 inhibitor (IRAP) from the medium conditioned by phorbol ester treated U937 cells and showed, on the basis of its sequence and properties, that this molecule is IL-1ra.

The structure of *IL-1ra* turned out to be very interesting in that it showed significant homology to *IL-1* (Fig. 1). The homologies are clustered rather than distributed, implying that they are important either for the structure of the molecule, or for its interactions with the receptor. This suggests that IL-1ra is the third member of the IL-1 class of molecules. This has been confirmed recently by the isolation of a genomic clone for IL-1ra showing that two of the

1 R-P-S-G-R-K-S-S-K-M-Q-A-F-R-I-W-D-V-N-Q

21 K-T-F-Y-L-R-N-N-Q-L-V-A-G-Y-L-Q-G-P-N-V

41 N-L-E-E-K-I-D-V-V-P-I-E-P-H-A-L-F-L-G-I

61 H-G-G-K-M-C-L-S-C-V-K-S-G-D-E-T-R-L-Q-L

81 E-A-V-N-I-T-D-L-S-E-N-R-K-Q-D-K-R-F-A-F

101 I-R-S-D-S-G-P-T-T-S-F-E-S-A-A-C-P-G-W-F

121 L-C-T-A-M-E-A-D-Q-P-V-S-L-T-N-M-P-D-E-G

141 V-M-V-T-K-F-Y-F-Q-E-D-E 152

Figure 1. Sequence of human interleukin-1 receptor antagonist. Shaded areas represent residues homologous with IL-1α or IL-1β.

three intron-exon junctions are in the same positions as those of IL-1α and IL-1β (Furutani et al., 1986; Clark et al., 1986; Eisenberg, et al., 1991).

The sequence of IL-1ra contains a single N-glycosylation site which explains the finding that monocytes make a number of species of this inhibitor which run differently on SDS-PAGE but can be converted to a single band by treatment with N-glycosidase (Hannum et al., 1990). One of the forms of the IL-1ra molecule is not glycosylated and this has the same affinity for the IL-1 receptor on EL4 cells as the glycosylated forms (Hannum et al., 1990). The existence of a natural, nonglycosylated form of IL-1ra provides the rationale for expression of the cDNA in *E. coli*. The protein prepared from *E. coli* is identical to the non-glycosylated form of the monocyte derived protein with the exception that it has an N-terminal methionine residue. Most of the work that we describe below was carried out with this recombinant protein.

IL-1ra Binds to, but Does not Activate the Type I IL-1 Receptor

Our results indicate that IL-1ra binds to the IL-1 receptor, but that it fails to induce an IL-1-like response (Hannum et al., 1990). Receptor binding of IL-1ra is quite easily demonstrated with biosynthetically radiolabelled IL-1ra using conditions similar to those previously described for the IL-1 binding assay (Kilian et al., 1986). Labelled IL-1ra is prevented from binding to the receptor equally well by IL-1ra, IL-1α and IL-1β, showing that the Type I IL-1 receptor of mouse EL4 cells has an affinity for IL-1ra that is very similar to its affinity for IL-1α and IL-1β (Fig. 2). A similar experiment demonstrated that IL-1ra also blocks the IL-1 receptor on human Hfl1 cells.

The finding that IL-1ra fails to activate the IL-1 receptor is a novel one in that no other natural protein *receptor antagonists* have yet been described. We have therefore explored quite intensively the validity of this finding. 'In view of the myriad actions of IL-1 *in vitro* it is extremely difficult to rule out the possibility of agonist activity in all cases. However, we have tested for agonist activity in several IL-1 assays *in vitro* and *in vivo* and have seen no response to IL-1ra

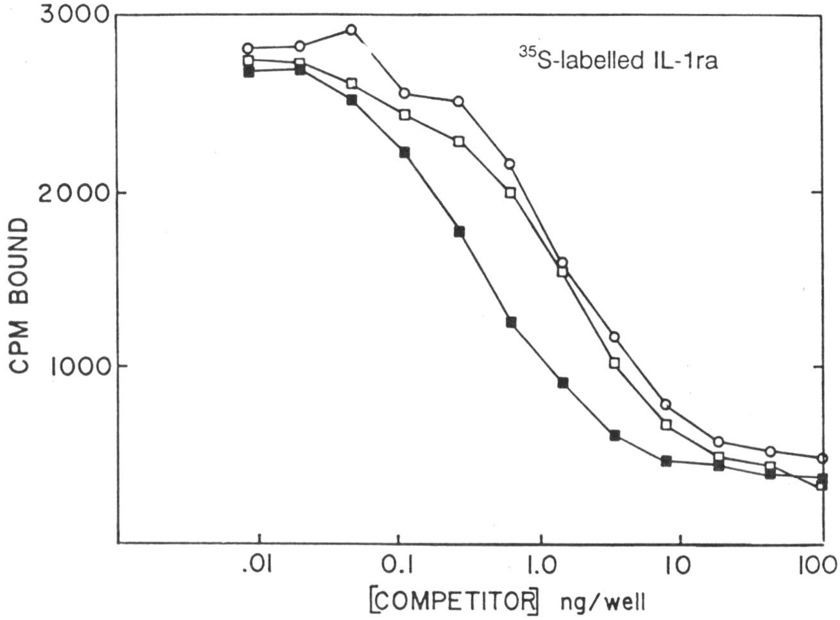

Figure 2. Receptor-competition assay in which ~1 ng ^{35}S-labelled antagonist was inhibited from binding to EL4-6.1 cells by varying amounts of cold recombinant IL-1α (■), IL-1β (○), and recombinant antagonist (□).

For example, we have shown that IL-1ra fails to activate fibroblasts for the synthesis of PGE2 at a concentration that is 100-fold above the effective concentration of IL-1 (Hannum et al., 1990; Arend et al., 1990), and that it fails to activate human umbilical vein endothelial cells for neutrophil binding at a concentration 10,000-fold higher than the effective concentration of IL-1 (Eisenberg et al., 1989; and manuscript in preparation).

To eliminate the need to demonstrate the antagonist nature of IL-1ra in all the many assays for IL-1 we have begun to explore the effects of IL-1ra on what are thought to be the initial, and presumably common steps of all IL-1 actions on cells. Two early events following the binding of IL-1 to cells are the induction of a protein kinase activity (Bird and Saklatvala, 1990) and the internalisation of the IL-1 · IL-1 receptor complex (Mizel et al., 1987). The protein kinase activity is easily assayed because it results in down modulation of the EGF receptor (Bird and Saklatvala, 1990). Preliminary tests of the activity of IL-1ra in this assay have shown that it fails to down modulate the EGF receptor at concentrations that are 10,000-fold higher than the effective concentration of IL-1 (Dripps et al., 1991). The internalisation of IL-1 can be assayed by the acid-stable association of IL-1 with cells. Preliminary studies of the fate of radiolabelled IL-1ra bound to EL4 cells indicate that IL-1ra is not internalised (Dripps et al., 1991).

All of the available evidence seems to indicate that IL-1ra is the first member of a new class of molecules which act as protein *receptor antagonists*. This has exciting implications for the regulation of a number of cytokine and protein hormone-induced responses and it is to be hoped that the structure of IL-1ra will give some clue to the features of the molecule that allow it to bind to a receptor without activating a biological response.

IL-1ra Blocks the Response to Exogenous IL-1 in Tissue Explants and in Animals

Exogenous IL-1 induces a number of proinflammatory events including the synthesis of degradative enzymes and the extravasation of neutrophils. Together with our collaborators we have tested the ability of IL-1ra to block both of these events.

IL-1 causes cartilage explants to digest their proteoglycans (Steinberg et al., 1979), presumably as a result of the elaboration of proteinases. Dave Carmichael and Chris Smith at Synergen have shown that a 10-fold excess of IL-1ra in the culture medium protects the tissue from this IL-1 mediated destruction (Carmichael et al., 1989). Intradermal injection of IL-1 into rabbits causes an accumulation of neutrophils at the site of injection (Cybulsky et al., 1986) and Myron Cybulsky has shown that injection of IL-1ra at the same site reduces this response (Cox et al., manuscript in preparation).

In addition to causing inflammation, IL-1 exerts a potent hypotensive effect on animals (Okusawa et al., 1988). Kjell Ohlsson and his colleagues have shown that this response can be abolished by doses of IL-1ra that are about 300-fold greater than the dose of IL-1 (Ohlsson et al., 1989, 1990).

In this case, and in the case of neutrophil extravasation, quite large excesses of IL-1ra over IL-1 are necessary to block its action. This is not a peculiarity of the animal experiments since similar effects are seen on cells and explants in culture (Eisenberg et al., 1990; Arend et al., 1990; Seckinger et al., 1990). We believe that the reason is related to the observation that only a very small proportion of the total IL-1 receptors needs to be occupied by IL-1 to elicit a physiological response (O'Neill et al., 1990), which is also the reason that IL-1 works at concentrations substantially below its Kd for the receptor.

IL-1ra as a Probe for the Role of IL-1 in Disease

The results described above lead us to believe that IL-1ra can be used as a probe to investigate the role of IL-1 in a number of diseases. There are already several examples of this use of the molecule as a result of our collaborations with academic investigators.

Fabio Cominelli and Charles Dinarello have established an impressive case for the role of IL-1 in an immune complex induced form of *ulcerative colitis*. The levels of IL-1 in inflamed colon tissue rise in parallel with the degree of inflammation and injury in the same fashion (Cominelli et al., 1990a). They have now provided conclusive evidence for this proposition using IL-1ra. IL-1ra injected into the rabbits two hours prior to the immune complexes and at various periods thereafter for 32 hours showed a dramatic effect in reducing several indices of inflammation, including ulceration of the colon (Cominelli et al., 1990b).

In collaboration with Kjell Ohlsson we have studied the role of IL-1 in *septic shock*. Some time ago Charles Dinarello and his colleagues showed that IL-1 could induce the hypotension associated with *septic shock* in rabbits and that IL-1 synergised with TNF in producing the organ necrosis that characterises this disease (Okusawa et al., 1988). To explore whether endogenous IL-1 plays an important role in septic shock we treated rabbits with a lethal dose of endotoxin and studied the effects of IL-1ra on mortality. 100 mg/kg delivered over the course of 24 hours reduced the mortality from 80% to 10% showing quite clearly that IL-1 plays a significant role in the mortality associated with this disease (Ohlsson et al., 1990). The IL-1ra treated animals who survived appeared to be in good health throughout the 7 day experiment.

One area of physiology where we have failed to demonstrate any effect of IL-1ra is the immune response. IL-1 is a comitogen for T-cells (Dinarello, 1989) and IL-1ra is able to block the proliferation of several TH2 cell clones *in vitro* (Chang et al., 1990). The first indication that IL-1ra would not act as an *immunosuppressant in vivo* came from toxicity studies in rats where anti IL-1ra antibodies were detected after 14 days of iv administration of the protein (Carmichael, personal communication). Subsequently, our colleagues at Roche have shown that IL-1ra has no effect on the DTH response, on the number of cytotoxic T-cells recovered from the spleen and popliteal lymph nodes of mice injected with allogeneic cells in the peritoneal cavity and the footpad respectively, or on the IgG and IgM responses in mice injected with KLH (Faherty et al., 1990). These results do not disprove the hypothesis that IL-1 is an essential component of the immune response since we may not have blocked IL-1 effects mediated by the Type II IL-1 receptor. However, they do raise questions about how IL-1 influences the immune response since IL-1ra should have blocked the Type 1 IL-1 receptor, which is normally found on T-cells.

In summary, IL-1ra shows every sign of being an important tool for probing IL-1 mediated events in pathophysiology. Thus far its usefulness has been confined to animal experiments. However, with the recent approval of an IND for the treatment of human rheumatoid arthritis patients with this drug we can look forward to answering the question of the role of IL-1 in human disease. Eventually we expect to be able to treat humans with IL-1ra, or derivatives of this protein, as a way of ameliorating IL-1 mediated disease.

Acknowledgements

We would like to thank our colleagues and collaborators for their contributions to the work described above and for permission to quote unpublished results.

References

Arend, W. P., Joslin, F. G. and Massoni, R. J. (1985). J. Immunol. 134: 3868–3875.

Arend W. P., Welgus, H. G., Thompson, R. C. and Eisenberg, S. P. (1990). J. Clin. Invest. 85: 1694–1697.

Balavoine, J-F., de Rochemonteix, B., Cruchaud, A. and Dayer, J-M. (1984). Lymphokine Research 3: 233.

Balavoine, J-F., de Rochemonteix, B., Williamson, K., Seckinger, P., Cruchaud, A. and Dayer, J-M. (1986). J. Clin. Invest. 78: 1120–1124.

Bird, T. A. and Saklatvala, J. (1990). J. Biol. Chem. 265: 235–240.

Carmichael, D. F., Smith, C. G. and Thompson, R. C. (1989). Cytokine 1: 89.

Carter, D. B., Deibel, M. R., Dunn, C. J., Tomich, C-S., Laborde, A. L., Slightom, J. L., Berger, A. E., Bienkowski, M. J., Sun, F. F., McEwan, R. N., Harris, P. K. W., Yem, A. W., Waszak, G. A., Chosay, J. G., Sieu, L. C., Hardee, M. M., Zurcher-Neely, H. A., Reardon, I. M., Heinrickson, R. L., Truesdell, S. E., Shelly, J. A., Eessalu, T. E., Taylor, B. M. and Tracey, D. E. (1990). Nature 344: 633–638.

Chang, T., Shea, C. M., Urioste, S., Thompson, R. C., Boom, W. H. and Abbas, A. K. (1990). J. Immunol. 145: 2803–2808.

Chizzonite, R., Truitt, T., Kilian, P. L., Stern, A. S., Nunes, P., Parker, K. P., Kaffka, K. L., Chua, A. O., Lugg, D. K. and Gubler, U. (1989). Proc. Nat. Acad. Sci. USA 86: 8029–8033.

Clark, B. D., Collins, K. L., Gands, M. S., Webb, A. C. and Auron, P. E. (1986). Nucl. Acids. Res. 14: 7897–7914.

Cominelli, F., Nast, C. C., Schindler, R., Clark, B., Llerena, R., Eysselein, V. E. and Dinarello, C. A. (1990a). Gastroenterology 98: A442.

Cominelli, F., Nast, C. C., Clark, B. D., Schindler, R., Llerena, R., Eysselein, V. E., Thompson, R. C. and Dinarello, C. A. (1990b). J. Clin. Invest. 86: 972–980.

Cybulsky, M. I., Colditz, I. G. and Movat, H. Z. (1986). Amer. J. Pathol. 124: 367–372.

Dinarello, C. A. (1989). Adv. Immunol. 44: 153–205.

Dripps, D. J., Brandhuber, B. J., Thompson, R. C., and Eisenberg, S. P. (1991) J. Biol. Chem. 266: 10331–10336.

Eisenberg, S. P., Brewer, M. T., Verderber, E., Heimdal, P., and Thompson, R. C. (1991) Proc. Natl. Acad. Sci. USA 88: 5232–5236.

Eisenberg, S. P., Evans, R. J., Arend, W. P., Verderber, E., Brewer, M. T., Hannum, C. H. and Thompson, R. C. (1990). Nature 343: 341–346.

Eisenberg, S. P., Thompson, R. C. and Cox, G. N. (1989). Cytokine 1: 90.

Faherty, D., Claudy, V., Plocinski, J. W., Chizzonite, R. and Benjamin, W. R. (1990). Inflammation Research Association, Fifth International Conference, Abstract No. 64.

Furutani, Y., Notake, M., Fukui, T., Ohue, M., Nomura, H., Yamada, M. and Nakamura, S. (1986). Nucl. Acids Res. 14: 3167–3179.

Hannum, C. H., Wilcox, C. J., Arend, W. P., Joslin, F. G., Dripps, D. J., Heimdal, P. L., Armes, L. G., Sommer, A., Eisenberg, S. P. and Thompson, R. C. (1990). Nature 343: 336–340.

Kilian, P. L., Kaffka, K. L., Stern, A. S., Woehle, D., Benjamin, W. R., Dechiara, T. M., Gubler, U., Farrar, J. J., Mizel, S. B. and Lomedico, P. T. (1986). J. Immunol. 136: 4509–4514.

Mizel, S. B., Kilian, P. L., Lewis, J. C., Paganelli, K. A. and Chizzonite, R. A. (1987). J. Immunol. 138: 2906–2912.

Ohlsson, K., Björk, P., Bergenfeldt, M., Eisenberg, S. P., Childs, J., Hannum, C. H. and Thompson, R. C. (1989). Cytokine 1: 131.

Ohlsson, K., Björk, P., Bergenfeldt, M., Hageman, R. and Thompson, R. C. (1990). Nature, 348: 550–552.

Okusawa, S., Gelfand, J. A., Ikejima, T., Connolly, R. J. and Dinarello, C. A. (1988). J. Clin. Invest. 81: 1162–1172.

O'Neill, L. A. J., Bird, T. A., Gearing, A. J. H. and Saklatvala, J. (1990). J. Biol. Chem. 265: 3146–3152.

Seckinger, P., Lowenthal, J. W., Williamson, K., Dayer, J-M. and MacDonald, H. R. (1987). J. Immunol. 139: 1546–1549.

Seckinger, P., Klein-Nulend, J., Alander, C., Thompson, R. C., Dayer, J-M. and Raisz, L. G. (1990). J. Immunol., 145: 4181–4184.

Sims, J. E., March, C. J., Cosman, D., Widmer, M. B., MacDonald, H. R., McMahon, C. J., Grubin, C. E., Wignall, J. M., Jackson, J. L., Call, S. M., Friend, D., Alpert, A. R., Gillis, S., Urdal, D. L. and Dower, S. K. (1988). Science 241: 585–589.

Steinberg, J., Sledge, C. B., Nobel, J. and Stirrat, C. R. (1979). Biochem. J. 180: 403–412.

AAS 35
Progress in Inflammation
Research and Therapy

Soluble and Cell Surface Receptors for Tumor Necrosis Factor

D. Wallach, H. Engelmann, Y. Nophar, D. Aderka[1], O. Kemper, V. Hornik, H. Holtmann[2] and C. Brakebusch[2]

Department of Molecular Genetics and Virology, The Weizmann Institute of Science, Rehovot, Israel 76100, [1]Department of Medicine T, Ichilov Hospital, Tel Aviv Medical Center, Tel Aviv, Israel and [2]School of Medicine, Hannover, FRG

Summary

Tumor necrosis factor (TNF) initiates its multiple effects on cell function by binding at a high affinity to specific cell surface receptors. Two different molecular species of these receptors, which are expressed differentially in different cells, have been identified. The cDNAs of both receptors have recently been cloned. Antibodies to one of these receptor species (the p55, type I receptor) can trigger a variety of TNF like effects by cross-linking of the receptor molecules. Thus, it is not TNF itself but its receptors that provide the signal for the response to this cytokine. The intracellular domains of the two receptors differ in structure, suggesting that they mediate different activities. Their extracellular domains, however, are structurally related. Both contain cysteine-rich repeats which are homologous to repeated structures found in the extracellular domains of the nerve growth factor receptor and the CDw40 protein. Truncated soluble forms of the two receptors, corresponding to these cysteine-rich repeated structures, have been detected in human urine and were later found to be present also in the serum. The serum levels of those soluble TNF receptors increase dramatically in certain pathological situations. Release of the soluble receptors from the cells seems to occur by proteolytic cleavage of the cell surface forms and appears to be a way of down-regulating the cell response to TNF. Because of their ability to bind TNF, the soluble receptors exert an inhibitory effect on TNF function, and may thus act as physiological attenuators of its activity.

Tumor necrosis factor (TNF), a polypeptide cytokine, produced primarily by mononuclear phagocytes, exerts effects on cell function which are involved in immune defense against a variety of different pathogenic agents. In certain diseases, however, TNF may itself become pathogenic. It is this later function of TNF that has attracted so much attention, recently, to this cytokine (Beutler and Cerami, 1988; Old, 1988).

Although its existence has already been known for quite some time (Granger and Kolb, 1968; Ruddle and Waksman, 1968; Carswell et al., 1975), it is only a few years since TNF was isolated (Aggarwal et al., 1985; Haranaka et al., 1985; Beutler et al., 1985a; Hahn et al., 1985). Information on the molecular basis for its function is therefore still limited. Shortly after its isolation it was shown in a number of laboratories that TNF binds with high affinity to specific receptors, which are expressed by a variety of cells (Baglioni et al., 1985; Beutler et al., 1985a; Kull et al., 1985; Tsujimoto et al., 1985; Aggarwal et al., 1986; Israel et al., 1986). On the basis of this finding it could already be surmised that TNF was not, as previously suspected, a "killer" molecule having an intrinsic toxic activity, but a cytokine, and that as in the case of other cytokines, it is not TNF itself but its receptors that provide the signal for the cellular response. It took several more years, however, for the receptors to be isolated, which made it possible to obtain formal evidence for this notion and to approach the study of the intracellular signals triggered by the receptors. As in the purification of TNF itself, the isolation of its receptors was hampered by the low abundancy of these molecules. Although these receptors are present in almost all cells, their amounts are very low, usually in the range of a few thousands of molecules per cell. Even more limiting, however, were difficulties arising out of the fact that these proteins are membrane-associated. Because of certain characteristics of the TNF molecule itself, the usual methods employed in the isolation of membranous proteins from detergent extracts of cells were not easily applicable here. Since these receptors exist in nature also in soluble forms, it is not surprising that in more than one laboratory the isolation of these soluble forms was achieved first, paving the way to the isolation of the membranous receptors.

Identification of Two TNF-Binding Proteins Present in Human Urine as Soluble Forms of Two Molecular Species of the Cell Surface TNF Receptors

A number of studies have shown that proteins of human urine exert a marked inhibitory effect on the *in vitro* function of TNF. Attempts to identify the proteins having this activity led to the successive isolation of two minor urinary proteins with TNF binding activity. These TNF-binding proteins (which we termed TBPI and TBPII) are similar in size (about 30,000) yet distinct immunologically (Engelmann et al., 1989, 1990a,b; Olsson et al., 1989; Seckinger et al., 1989).

Antibodies against both proteins inhibited the binding of TNF to cells. However their respective inhibitory capacities varied with the kind of cell examined (Engelmann et al., 1990a). This finding suggested that TBPI and TBPII cross-react immunologically with cell surface TNF receptors (TNF-Rs) of two different molecular species, which are expressed differentially in different cells. Indeed, further examination revealed that antibodies against TBPI immunoprecipitate a TNF-R of Mr 550000 (the type I or p55 receptor) from cell extracts, while antibodies to TBPII immunoprecipitate a receptor of Mr around 75000 (the type II or p75 receptor) (Engelmann et al., 1990b). The structural relationships between the two soluble TNF-binding proteins and their respective receptors were fully clarified after cloning of the cDNAs for the receptors (Loetscher et al., 1990; Schall et al., 1990; Nophar et al., 1990; Smith et al., 1990; Heller et al., 1990; Kohno et al., 1990). In some of the studied that led to the cloning, it was the knowledge of this structural relationship and of the structure of the soluble proteins which provided the basis for the cloning approach. Examination of the amino acid sequences in the receptors, disclosed by the cloning of their cDNAs, revealed that they contain sequences found in the soluble proteins. Recently we determined the full sequence of amino acids in one of the two TNF-binding proteins (TBPI) and found it to be completely matched by the sequence of amino acids in the extracellular domain of the immunologically cross reacting cell surface receptor (the type I, p55 receptor). Although the extracellular domains of the two TNF-Rs have non-identical amino acid sequences, as would be expected from their failure to cross-react immunologically, their structure is highly homologous. Both contain conserved cysteine-rich repeat structures which extend over almost their entire length. The extracellular domains of two other known receptors – the receptor for the nerve growth factor and the B-cell-activating antigen, CDw40 – also contain this conserved repetitive structure.

The cysteine-rich repeat structures extend over almost the whole length of the soluble urine-derived TNF binding proteins (Nophar et al., 1990).

Use of Antibodies Against the Extracellular Domains of the TNF-Rs to Explore Their Mode of Action

A number of receptor-mediated effects can be mimicked by cross-linking of the relevant receptors. Similarly, effects which are characteristic of TNF could be induced in cells by antibodies against the extracellular domain of the type I TNF-R (Engelmann et al., 1990b; Espevik et al., 1990). This mimetic effect of the antibodies was not due to their ability to present to cells a molecular structure identical with that of TNF. A comparative study of the ability of various antibodies against the receptor to mimic the activity of TNF indicated that this activity is due merely to their ability to cross-link the receptors (Engelmann et al., 1990b). This finding demonstrated conclusively that it is not TNF itself but its receptors that provide the signal for the cellular response. It also raised the possibility that aggregation of the TNF-Rs occurs also upon their activation by TNF, a notion which seems further supported by the fact that the TNF molecule itself is an oligomer and loses bioactivity upon dissociation to its monomeric form.

There is still no information on the nature of the biochemical signals which the TNF-Rs provide. Rapidly induced phosphorylation of certain proteins, such as HSP27, observed in cells treated with TNF, may provide a clue to the identity of such signals. Although these effects can also be triggered by cross-linking with the type I TNF-R molecules (Nophar et al., 1990), the sequence of amino acids in the intracellular domains of the two TNF-Rs indicate that neither of the two receptor species possesses intrinsic kinase activity, suggesting the involvement of additional cellular components, perhaps receptor associated proteins, in providing the signals. Since there is no apparent structural similarity between the intracellular domains of the two species of TNF-R, it seems likely that there are differences in the signals which they provide as well as in their effects. Conceivably, the effect of the two receptors are cell specific, to the extent that the receptors themselves are.

Physiological Significance of the Soluble Forms of the TNF-Rs

Does the interaction of TNF with the soluble TNF-Rs significantly affect the *in vivo* function of this cytokine as it does *in vitro*? Evaluation of the physiological significance of an extracellular factor can be achieved only by studies carried out at the level of the whole organism, and therefore presents far greater difficulties than an evaluation of the function of a cell-associated component such as the cell surface TNF-Rs. Our present notions of the *in vivo* function of the soluble TNF-Rs can be based only on indirect information, such as knowledge of the kinds of situations in which the formation of these proteins occur and the nature of the mechanisms involved in this process.

ELISA tests for the determination of the serum levels of the two soluble TNF-Rs have revealed that both proteins are present in normal sera, though in low amounts, and that their serum levels increase dramatically in certain pathological states. The range of diseases in which such an increase occurs is very wide and includes numerous autoimmune diseases, infectious diseases and other inflammatory processes. Interestingly, both types of soluble receptors are increased also in the sera of patients with solid tumors or hematological malignancies. The incidence of such increase in cancer patients is rather high, exceeding even the incidence of increase of the carcinoembryonic antigen, one of the most widely used diagnostic parameters for cancer (Aderka et al., 1991). At least part of this increase may reflect shedding of the TNF-Rs by the tumor cells themselves. Indeed, we found continuous production of the soluble TNF-Rs in culture by cells of various tumor-derived lines. In normal cells, however, formation of the soluble TNF-Rs seems to be largely dependent on stimulation of the cells. The rapidity with which this process occurs in response to certain stimuli, as well as the absence of any detectable amounts of soluble TNF-Rs within cells, suggests that it reflects cleavage of the existing cell surface receptors, not *de novo* formation of the soluble receptors, by a mechanism independent of the formation of the membranous forms (Porteu and Nathan, 1990, Lantz et al., 1990). Consistently, it was found that in CHO cells transfected with cDNA for the type I TNF-R, the cDNA encodes both the cell surface and the soluble forms of the receptor

(Nophar et al., 1990). Activation of such a process of cleavage may result in a significant decrease in the amounts of cell surface TNF-Rs, and may thus represent a mode of down regulation of the response to TNF. In some of the pathological situations in which TNF may cause harm this process seems to occur at an increased rate, as reflected in significantly increased levels of soluble TNF-Rs in the sera of patients with those diseases. The concentrations of soluble receptors obtained in such cases are high enough to exert an inhibitory effect on TNF function *in vitro*, (unpublished data). It remains to be determined whether such inhibition is a significant factor in the *in vivo* response to TNF in these cases, and whether it can be further augmented by injecting patients with a higher dose of the soluble receptors.

Acknowledgements

Research in the author's laboratory was supported by grants from Inter-Lab Ltd., Ness-Ziona, Israel, as well as by grant from the National Council for Research and Development, Israel, and the German Cancer Research Center.

References

Aderka, D., Engelmann, H., Hornik, V., Skornick, Y., Yoram, L., Wallach, D., and Kushtai, G., (1991) Cancer res. (in press).

Aggarwal, B. B., Eessalu, T. E. and Hass, P. E. (1986). Nature 328: 665–667.

Aggarwal, B. B., Kohr, W. J., Hass, P. E., Moffat, B., Spencer, S. A., Henzel, W. J., Bringman, T. S., Nedwin, G. E., Goeddel, D. V. and Harkins, R. N. (1985). J. Biol. Chem. 260: 2345–2354.

Baglioni, C., McCandless, S., Tavernier, J. and Fiers, W. (1985) J. Biol. Mech. 260: 13395–13397.

Beutler, B., Greenwald, D., Hulmes, J. D., Chang, M., Pan, Y.-C. E., Mathison, J., Ulevich, R. and Cerami, A. (1985a). Nature 316: 552–554.

Beutler, B. A., Mahoney, J., Le Trang, N., Pekala, P. and Cerami, A. (1985b). J. Exp. Med. 161: 984–995.

Beutler, B. and Cerami, A. (1988). Annu. Rev. Biochem. 57: 505–518.

Carswell, E. A., Old, L. J., Kassel, R. L., Green, S., Fiore, N. and Williamson, B. (1975). Proc. Natl. Acad. Sci. USA 72: 3666–3670.

Engelmann, H., Aderka, D., Rubinstein, M., Rotman, D. and Wallach D. (1989). J. Biol. Chem. 264: 11974–11980.

Engelmann, H., Novick, D., and Wallach, D. (1990a). J. Biol. Chem. 265: 1531–1536.

Engelmann, H., Holtmann, H., Brakebusch, C., Shemer-Avni, Y., Sarov, I., Nophar, Y., Hadas, E., Leitner, O. and Wallach, D. (1990b). J. Biol. Chem. 265: 14479–14484.

Espevik, T., Brockhaus, M., Loetscher, H., Nonstad, U. and Shalaby, R. (1990). J. Exp. Med. 171: 415–426.

Granger, G. A. and Kolb, W. P. (1968). J. Immunol. 101: 111–120.

Hahn, T., Toker, L., Budilovsky, S., Aderka, D., Eshhar, Z. and Wallach, D. (1985). Proc. Natl. Acad. Sci. USA. 82: 3814–3818.

Haranaka, K., Satomi, N., Sakurai, A. and Nariuchi, H. (1985). Int. J. Cancer 36: 395–400.

Heller, R. A., Song, K., Onasch, M. A., Fischer, W. H., Chang, D. and Ringold, G. M. (1990). Proc. Natl. Acad. Sci. USA. 87: 6151–6155.

Israel, S., Hahn, T., Holtmann, H. and Wallach, D. (1986). Immunol. Lett. 12: 217–224.

Kohno, T., Brewer, M. T., Baker, S. L., Schwarts, P. E., King, M. W., Hale, K. K., Squires, C. H., Thompson, R. C. and Vannice, J. L. (1990). Proc. Natl. Acad. Sci. USA, in press.

Kull, F. C. Jr., Jacobs, S. and Cuatrecasas, P. (1985). Proc. Natl. Acad. Sci. USA 82: 5756–5760.

Lantz, M., Gulberg, U., Nilsson, E. and Olsson, I. (1990). J. Clin. Invest., in press.

Loetscher, H., Pan, Y-C. E., Lahm, H-W., Gentz, R., Brockhaus, M., Tabuchi, H. and Lesslauer, W. (1990). Cell 61: 351–359.

Nophar, Y., Kemper, O., Brakebusch, C., Engelmann, H., Zwang, R., Aderka, D., Holtmann, H. and Wallach, D. (1990). EMBO J. 9: 3269–3278.

Old, L. R. (1988). Sci. Am. 258: 41–49.

Olsson, I., Lantz, M., Nilsson, E., Peetre, C., Thysell, H., Grubb, A. and Adolf, G. (1989). Eur. J. Haematol. 42: 270–275.

Porteu, F. and Nathan, C. (1990). J. Exp. Med. 172: 599–607.

Ruddle, N. and Waksman, B. H. (1968). J. Exp. Med. 128: 1267–1279.

Seckinger, P., Isaaz, S., and Dayer, J-M. (1989). J. Biol. Chem. 264: 11966–11973.

Schall, T. J., Lewis, M., Koller, K. J., Lee, A., Rice, G. C., Wong, G. H. W., Gatanaga, T., Granger, G. A., Lentz, R., Raab, H., Kohr, W. J. and Goeddel, D. V. (1990). Cell 61: 361–370.

Smith, C. A., Davis, T., Anderson, D., Solam, L., Beckmann, M. P., Jerzy, R., Kower, S. K., Cosman, D. and Goodwin, R. G. (1990). Science 248: 1019–1023.

Tsujimoto, M., Yip, Y. K. and Vilcek, J. (1985). Proc. Natl. Acad. Sci. USA. 82: 7626–7630.

Wallach, D., Aderka, D., Engelmann, H., Nophar, Y., Kemper, O., Holtmann, H., Brakebusch, C., Villa, S., Grossi Gondi, F., and Bucciarelli, U., (1991) in: Proceedings of the 3rd International TNF conference (T. Osawa and B. Bonavida eds.) S. Karger, Basel. (in press).

Proteinases & Tissue Destruction

AAS 35
Progress in Inflammation
Research and Therapy

Stromelysin: Structure and Function

H. G. Welgus
Division of Dermatology, Jewish Hospital at Washington University Medical Center, 216 South Kingshighway, St. Louis, MO 63110, USA

Summary

Stromelysin, a member of the metalloproteinase gene family, may play a crucial role in pathological turnover of connective tissues. The following manuscript will review structural features and functional properties of stromelysin and its related proteinases.

Stromelysin, also referred to as transin and MMP-3, is an important member of the metalloproteinase gene family. Initially called "proteoglycanase," the enzyme is known to cleave a variety of extracellular matrix substrates including proteoglycans, laminin, fibronectin, native collagen types IV and IX (non-helical domains only), the propeptides of native type I procollagen, and denatured collagens of all genetic types (Wilhelm et al., 1987; Baricos et al., 1988., Bejarano et al., 1988; Nguyen et al., 1989; Okada et al., 1989). Matrix components resistant to catalysis by stromelysin include native *helical* collagens and elastin (Senior et al., 1990). Furthermore, stromelysin has been shown to participate in the activation of interstitial collagenase by cleavage of a 2 kDa fragment from the trypsin-activated enzyme (Murphy et al., 1987; Ito & Nagase, 1988; He et al., 1989). This additional cleavage confers an 8-fold enhanced catalytic activity as compared to trypsin-activated collagenase (He et al., 1989).

Stromelysin is secreted as zymogen species of 60 and 57 kDa. The protein component of these forms is identical, and the zymogens differ only in glycosylation of the higher molecular weight species (Wilhelm et al., 1987). Prostromelysin fails to bind susceptible substrates or to interact with TIMP. Capacity for these functions is achieved only following activation of the zymogen species. Activation can be accomplished in the laboratory either proteolytically or by the addition of organomercurial compounds. Physiologic mechanisms of activation are only speculative. Proteinases capable of activating prostromelysin include trypsin, plasmin, kallikrein, neutrophil elastase, cathepsin-G, and mast cell tryptase (Gruber et al., 1989; Okada and Nakanishi, 1989; Nagase et al., 1990). These enzymes cleave within a susceptible region of prostromelysin involving residues Phe^{34}-Asp^{39}. The organomercurials induce an intramolecular autocatalysis at residues Glu^{68}-Val^{69}. Thus, exposure to either proteinases or organomercurials results in conversion of prostromelysin to intermediate forms of 46–53 kDa (Nagase et al., 1990). These intermediates undergo a bimolecular reaction to generate the stable 45 kDa active stromelysin form. This latter process is concentration-dependent. Furthermore, the 45 kDa active species can be autocatalyzed to a 28 kDa form lacking the C-terminal region, yet retaining full catalytic activity (Nagase et al., 1990).

Stromelysin is produced by a relatively limited number of cell types that include fibroblasts and mononuclear phagocytes (Wilhelm et al., 1987; Welgus et al., 1990). In the case of mononuclear phagocytes, capacity for stromelysin production is dependent upon cell differentiation. Of all the metalloproteinases secreted by mononuclear phagocytes, stromelysin requires the most differentiated phenotype for expression. Monocytes lack capacity to produce stromelysin; only the fully differentiated and LPS-stimulated macrophage is capable of its secretion (Welgus et al., 1990). On a per cell basis, stimulated macrophages produce 10% of the stromelysin as stimulated fibroblasts (Welgus et al., 1990).

Production of stromelysin is highly regulatable by a variety of physiologic and pharmacologic agents. Thus far, all regulatory factors have been shown to function by transcriptional mechanisms (Frisch et al., 1987; Kerr et al., 1988; Machida et al., 1988; Quinones et al., 1989). Stimulation of stromelysin biosynthesis is observed in response to certain cytokines including IL-1 and TNF (Frisch et al., 1987; Quinones et al., 1989). Growth factors, including EGF and PDGF, also upregulate its expression (Matrisian et al., 1986; Kerr et al., 1988a; Kerr et al., 1988b; Machida et al., 1988; McDonnell et al., 1990). In a series of elegant studies (Kerr et al., 1988a; McDonnell et al., 1990), Matresian and colleagues have shown that EGF stimulates stromelysin production by a *c-fos*-independent mechanism and PDGF by a *c-fos*-dependent process. Furthermore, TGF-β blocks EGF induction of stromelysin (Kerr et al., 1988b; Machida et al., 1988). Expression of stromelysin is also enhanced by oncogenic viruses including polyoma and Rous sarcoma, by the cellular H-ras oncogene, and by phorbol esters (Chin et al., 1985; Matrisian et al., 1986a; Breathnach et al., 1987; Frisch et al., 1987; Kerr et al., 1988b). Cytochalasins that disrupt cellular architecture stimulate stromelysin release (Breathnach et al., 1987). Recently, Werb and colleagues (Werb et al., 1989) have shown that occupancy of $\alpha_5\beta_1$ integrin receptors induces a parallel stimulation of fibroblast collagenase and stromelysin production. Finally, Brinckerhoff has demonstrated co-induction of collagenase and stromelysin following heat shock of cells (Vance et al, 1989).

Cytokine or growth factor-induced stromelysin production can be ablated by certain agents. As mentioned previously, TGF-β blocks EGF induction of this proteinase (Kerr et al., 1988b; Machida et al., 1988). Dexamethasone and retinoid compounds, potent suppressors of a variety of metalloproteinases (Frisch and Ruley, 1987; Okada et al., 1988), also inhibit stromelysin biosynthesis. Recently, we have shown that gamma-interferon potently suppresses LPS-induced collagenase and stromelysin production in macrophages (Shapiro et al., 1990). Interestingly, the lymphokine failed to affect production of 92 kDa type IV collagenase or TIMP.

Two other stromelysin-related proteinases have recently been described. These are designated stromelysin-2 (Breathnach et al., 1987; Muller et al., 1988; Nicholson et al., 1989; Quantin et al., 1989) and PUMP (Quantin et al., 1989). Stromelysin-2 is very similar to stromelysin-1 in exon/intron structure of the genes (Breathnach et al., 1987). In one stretch of >400 bases, there is 98% homology. However, overall, stromelysin-1 and stromelysin-2 are 71% homologous in amino acid sequence (Breathnach et al., 1987). Both proteins are induced by phorbol esters and both have similar substrate specificities. Furthermore, both can participate in the activation of interstitial procollagenase, although stromelysin-1 is more effective. However, very significant differences exist between these two highly related proteinases. The promoter regions of stromelysin-1 and stromelysin-2 are quite different (Breathnach et al., 1987). As a consequence, only stromelysin-1 is induced by EGF, IL-1, and the cytochalasins. Thus, it is possible that both proteinases may function in a catalytically similar manner, but are regulated by different inducing stimuli and perhaps even produced by different cell types.

PUMP or "putative metalloproteinase" is much less related to stromelysin-1 than is stromelysin-2. Nevertheless, PUMP was initially isolated during the cloning of stromelysin under low stringency conditions (Muller et al, 1988; Quantin et al, 1989). PUMP contains the amino-terminal domain common to all metalloproteinases and the zinc-binding catalytic site. It lacks the C-terminal hemopexin (and vitronectin)-like domain of metalloenzymes and is thus approximately half the molecular weight of the other proteinases. Interestingly, PUMP is similar to the overprocessed 28 kDa active stromelysin species. PUMP is secreted in a zymogen form, is TIMP-inhibitable, and cleaves casein, fibronectin, and gelatin (Quantin et al. 1989).

Many studies suggest that stromelysin plays a critical role in abnormal biologic processes including the inflammatory arthritides and tumor invasion. It is the only metalloproteinase capable of degrading proteoglycans, attacking both core and link proteins (Gunja-Smith et al., 1989; Nguyen et al., 1989). Furthermore, it seems likely that stromelysin is involved in tumor progression, as suggested by Matresian and colleagues (Matrisian et al., 1986b) who have shown higher enzyme mRNA levels in squamous carcinomas as compared to benign papillomas. Stromelysin mRNA levels also correlate positively with increasing aggressiveness of metastatic neoplasms. The next several years should uncover additional new information regarding the role of stromelysin and its related preteinases in these important biologic processes.

References

Baricos, W. H., Murphy, G., Zhou, Y., Nguyen, H. H. and Shah, S. V. (1988). Degradation of glomerular basement membrane by purified mammalian metalloproteinases. Biochem. J. 254: 609–612.

Bejarano, P. A., Noelken, M. E., Suzuki, K., Hudson, B. G. and Nagase, H. (1988). Degradation of basement membranes by human matrix metalloproteinase 3 (stromelysin). Biochem. J. 256: 413–419.

Breathnach, R., Matrisian, L. M., Gesnel, M.-C., Staub, A. and Leroy, P. (1987). Sequences coding for part of oncogene-induced transin are highly conserved in a related rat gene. Nuc. Ac. Res. 15: 1139–1151.

Chin, J. R., Murphy, G. and Werb, Z. (1985). Stromelysin, a connective tissue-degrading metalloendopeptidase secreted by stimulated rabbit synovial fibroblasts in parallel with collagenase. J. Biol. Chem. 260: 12367–12376.

Frisch, S. M., Clark, E. J. and Werb, Z. (1987). Coordinate regulation of stromelysin and collagenase genes determined with cDNA probes. Proc. Natl. Acad. Sci. USA. 84: 2600–2604.

Frisch, S. M. and Ruley, H. E. (1987). Transcription from the stromelysin promoter is induced by interleukin-1 and repressed by dexamethasone. J. Biol. Chem. 262: 16300–16304.

Gruber, B. L., Marchese, M. J., Suzuki, K., Schwartz, L. B., Okada, Y., Nagase, H. and Ramamurthy, N. S. (1989). Synovial procollagenase activation by human mast cell tryptase: dependence upon matrix metalloproteinase 3 activation. J. Clin. Invest. 84: 1657–1662.

Gunja-Smith, Z., Nagase, H. and Woessner, J. F. Jr. (1989). Purification of the neutral proteoglycan-degrading metalloproteinase from human articular cartilage tissue and its identification as stromelysin matrix metalloproteinase-3. Biochem. J. 258: 115–119.

He, C., Wilhelm, S. M., Pentland, A. P., Marmer, B. L., Grant G. A., Eilsen, A. Z. and Goldberg, G. I. (1989). Tissue cooperation in a proteolytic cascade activating human interstitial collagenase. Proc. Natl. Acad. Sci. USA. 86: 2632–2636.

Ito, A. and Nagase, H. (1988). Evidence that human rheumatoid synovial matrix metalloproteinase 3 is an endogenous activator of procollagenase. Arch. Biochem. Biophys. 267: 211–216.

Kerr, L. D., Holt, J. T. and Matrisian, L. M. (1988a). Growth factors regulate transin gene expression by *c-fos*-dependent and *c-fos*-independent pathways. Science. 242: 1424–1427.

Kerr, L. D., Olashaw, N. E. and Matrisian, L. M. (1988b). Transforming growth factor $\beta 1$ and cAMP inhibit transcription of epidermal growth factor- and oncogene-induced transin RNA. J. Biol. Chem. 263: 16999–17005.

Machida, C. M., Muldoon, L. L., Rodland, K. D. and Magun, B. E. (1988). Transcriptional modulation of transin gene expression by epidermal growth factor and transforming growth factor beta. Mol. Cell. Biol. 8: 2479–2483.

Matrisian, L. M., Bowden, G. T., Krieg, P., Furstenberger, G., Briand, J.-P., Leroy P. and Breathnach, R. (1986b). The mRNA coding for the secreted protease transin is expressed more abundantly in malignant than in benign tumors. Proc. Natl. Acad. Sci. USA. 83: 9413–9417.

Matrisian, L. M., Leroy, P., Ruhlmann, C., Gesnel, M.-C. and Breathnach, R. (1986a). Isolation of the oncogene and epidermal growth factor-induced transin gene: Complex control in rat fibroblasts. Mol. Cell. Biol. 6: 1676–1686.

McDonnell, S. E., Kerr, L. D. and Matrisian, L. M. (1990). Epidermal growth factor stimulation of stromelysin mRNA in rat fibroblasts requires induction of proto-oncogenes *c-fos* and *c-jun* and activation of protein kinase C. Mol. Cell. Biol. 10: 4284–4293.

Muller, D., Quantin, B., Gesnel, M. C., Millon-Collard, R., Abecasses, J. and Breathnach, R. (1988). Collagenase gene family in humans consists of at least four members. Biochem. J. 253: 187–192.

Murphy, G., Cockett, M. I., Stephens, P. E., Smith, B. J. and Docherty, A. J. P. (1987). Stromelysin is an activator of procollagenase. Biochem. J. 248: 265–268.

Nagase, H., Enghild, J. J., Suzuki, K. and Salvesen, G. (1990). Stepwise activation mechanisms of the precursor of matrix metalloproteinase 3 (stromelysin) by proteinases and (4-aminophenyl) mercuric acetate. Biochemistry 29: 5783–5789.

Nguyen, Q., Murphy, G,. Roughley, P. J. and Mort. J. S. (1989). Degradation of proteoglycan aggregate by a cartilate metalloproteinase. Biochem. J. 259: 61–67.

Nicholson, R., Murphy, G. and Breathnach, R. (1989). Human and rat malignant-tumor-associated mRNAs encode stromelysin-like-metalloproteinases. Biochemistry 28: 5195–5203.

Okada, Y., Harris, E. D. Jr. and Nagase, H. (1988). The precursor of a metallo-endopeptidase from human rheumatoid synovial fibroblasts. Biochem. J. 254: 731–741.

Okada, Y., Konomi, H., Yada, T., Kimata, K. and Nagase, H. (1989). Degradation of type IX collagen by matrix metalloproteinase 3 (stromelysin) from human rheumatoid synovial cells. FEBS Let. 244: 473–476.

Okada, Y. and Nakanishi, I. (1989). Activation of matrix metalloproteinase 3 (stromelysin) and matrix metalloproteinase 2 ('gelatinase') by human neutrophil elastase and cathepsin-G. FEBS Let. 249: 353–356.

Quantin, B, Murphy, G. and Breathnach, R. (1989). Pump-1 cDNA codes for a protein with characteristics similar to those of classical collagenase family members. Biochemistry 28: 5327–5334.

Quinones, S., Saus, J., Otani, Y., Harris, E. D. Jr. and Kurkinen, M. (1989). Transcriptional regulation of human stromelysin. J. Biol. Chem. 264: 8339–8344.

Senior, R. M., Griffin, G. L., Fliszar, C. J., Shapiro, S. D., Goldberg, G. I. and Welgus, H. G. (1991). Human 92- and 72-kilodalton type IV collagenases are elastases. J. Biol. Chem. 266: 7870–7875.

Shapiro, S. D., Campbell, E. J., Kobayashi, D. K. and Welgus, H. G. (1990). Immune modulation of metalloproteinase production in human macrophages: Selective pre-translational suppression of interstitial collagenase and stromelysin biosynthesis by gamma interferon. J. Clin. Invest. 86: 1204–1210.

Vance, B. A., Kowalski, C. G. and Brinckerhoff, C. E. (1989). Heat shock of rabbit synovial fibroblasts increases expression of mRNAs for two metalloproteinases, collagenase and stromelysin. J. Cell Biol. 108: 2037–2043.

Welgus, H. G. (1991). Campbell, E. J., Cury, J. D., Eisen, A. Z., Senior, R. M., Wilhelm, S. M., and Goldberg, G. I. (1990). Neutral metalloproteinases produced by human mononuclear phagocytes: Enzyme profile, regulation and expression during cellular development. J. Clin. Invest. 86: 1496–1502.

Werb, Z., Tremble, P. M., Behrendtsen, O., Crowley, E. and Damsky, C. H. (1989). Signal transduction through the fibronectin receptor induces collagenase and stromelysin gene expression. J. Cell Biol. 109: 877–889.

Wilhelm, S. C., Collier, I. E., Kronberger, A., Eisen, A. Z., Marmer, B. L., Grant, G. A., Bauer, E. A. and Goldberg, G. I. (1987). Human skin fibroblast stromelysin: Structure, glycosylation, substrate specificity, and differential expression in normal and tumorigenic cells. Proc. Natl. Acad. Sci., USA. 84: 6725–6729.

AAS 35
Progress in Inflammation
Research and Therapy

The Regulation of Connective Tissue Metalloproteinases by Natural Inhibitors

G. Murphy

Strangeways Research Laboratory, Cambridge CB1 4RN, UK

Summary

The family of matrix metalloproteinases have a fundamental role in the breakdown of connective tissue matrices in both physiological and pathological processes. The endogenous levels of the tissue inhibitors of metalloproteinases are a key determinant in the regulation of the activity of these enzymes. Current research on the mode of action of these inhibitors at the molecular level, aimed at their use as models for low molecular weight inhibitors, is outlined. Preliminary evidence for inhibitor deficiency in disease states and their potential use as therapeutic agents are summarised.

Introduction

The matrix metalloproteinases (MMPs) are a family of zinc-dependent endopeptidases that have the combined ability to degrade the various components of connective tissue matrices. They are synthesised and secreted by connective tissue cells as well as some cells of haematopoietic origin and are known to be important both in normal remodelling processes and in the accelerated destruction occurring in many diseases. The regulation of MMPs is necessarily stringent, occurring not only at the level of gene expression but extracellularly, following secretion, by the action of activators of proenzyme forms and of inhibitors, which can also be modulated at several levels. Two major types of MMP inhibitor have been clearly identified, $\alpha 2$ macroglobulin and the tissue inhibitors of MMPs, TIMPs; less well defined inhibitors remain to be further analysed. This review will briefly outline our current knowledge about the TIMPs in relation to their role in connective tissue degradation.

Molecular Studies of TIMPs

Two forms of the MMP inhibitors, TIMPs, have been studied in detail. The major form TIMP-1 is an M_r 30000 glycoprotein and is synthesised by most connective tissue cells as well as macrophages; TIMP-1 resides in platelet α granules and can be identified in most body fluids (reviewed by Cawston, 1986). It specifically acts against the MMPs and has no activity against other metalloendopeptidases; it forms high affinity, non-covalent and essentially irreversible complexes with the active forms of the MMPs (Cawston et al., 1983; Welgus et al., 1985; Murphy et al., 1989). 1 mole of TIMP-1 binds 1 mole of MMP in all cases studied. Active TIMP-1 can be recovered from enzyme complexes (Murphy et al., 1989; Lefebvre and Vaes, 1989). It has recently been shown that TIMP-1 also binds to the pro form of M_r 95000 gelatinase (type IV collagenase; Wilhelm et al., 1989) although the physiological significance of this is not clear. The molecular mechanism of TIMP binding to active MMPs has not yet been elucidated. Welgus et al., (1985) carried out preliminary kinetic studies which indicated that TIMP-collagenase binding was non-competitive in nature. Pre-treatment of MMPs with the Zn^{2+} chelator 1,10 phenanthroline prevents complex formation (Galloway et al., 1983). Complex formation is slow and both active collagenase and stromelysin have been found to bind more rapidly to α_2-macroglobulin than to TIMP in mixtures of the two inhibitors (Cawston et al., 1986; Murphy et al., 1989).

A second, less abundant, but nonetheless ubiquitous form of TIMP, TIMP-2, has been isolated from a number of cell culture systems and tissue extracts. This inhibitor, M_r 23000, is largely unglycosylated, but current studies suggest that its properties are very similar to those of TIMP-1 in terms of binding to active MMPs, with the exception that TIMP-2 binds to the pro form of the M_r 72000 gelatinase (Stetler-Stevenson et al., 1989). The distribution of TIMP-2 is not well documented but it is notable that it has been isolated from articular cartilage extracts (Murray et al., 1986; Bunning et al., 1984).

Both TIMP-1 and TIMP-2 have been cloned from a number of species (Docherty et al., 1985; Carmichael et al., 1986; Boone et al., 1990). Although their overall primary sequence similarity is only

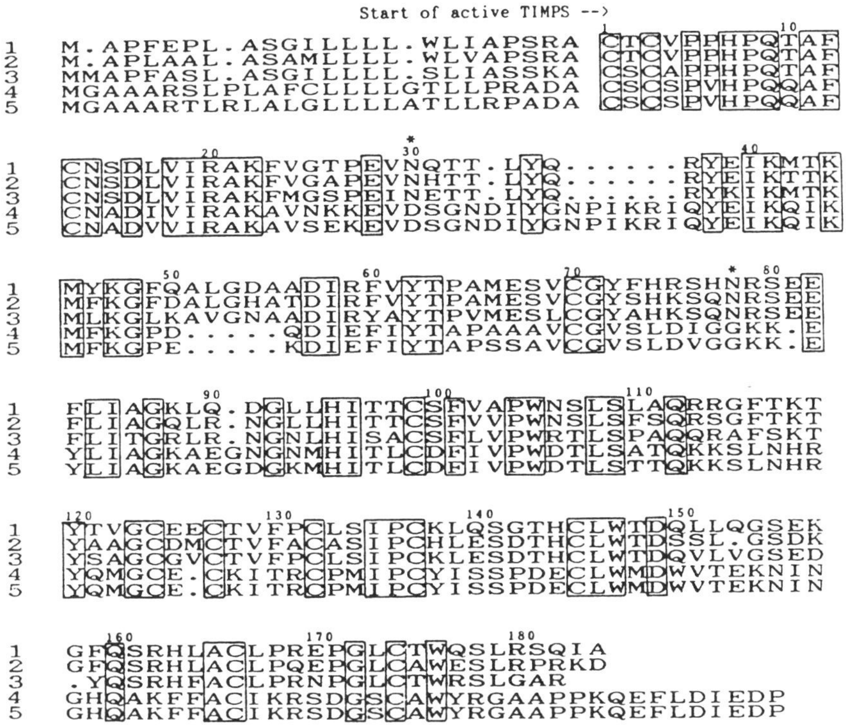

Figure 1. Alignment of the primary sequences of TIMP-1 and TIMP-2 from different species. The sequences are all deduced from their respective cDNAs. Identical residues are boxed and the two potential glycosylation sites in TIMP-1s are marked*. 1. Human TIMP-1 (numbered sequence; Docherty et al., 1985). 2. Rabbit TIMP-1 (Horowitz et al., 1989). 3. Mouse TIMP-1 (Edwards et al., 1986). 4. Bovine TIMP-2 (Boone et al., 1990). 5. Human TIMP-2 (Boone et al., 1990).

40%, it can be seen that the twelve cysteine residues are completely conserved, as are other key residues (Fig. 1). TIMP-1 has recently been shown to have six disulphide bonds which have been assigned as C_1-C_{70}, C_3-C_{99}, C_{13}-C_{124}, C_{127}-C_{174}, C_{132}-C_{137} and C_{145}-C_{166} (Williamson et al., 1990). It seems reasonable to assume that TIMP-2 will show a comparable disulphide bond structure. The intact structure is required for TIMP activity; reduction of the inhibitors abolishes their activity. Trypsin generated fragments of TIMP-1 have no activity (R. Williamson & G. Murphy, unpublished), neither do the N and C terminal halves of the molecule, expressed separately in an *in vitro* translation system (Coulombe & Skup, 1988). It is anticipated that further analyses of TIMP function will require detailed biochemical and recombinant DNA studies which analyse the role of specific residues and loops of the inhibitors. Because of the unique specificity of the TIMPs for the MMPs, this will yield important information for the design of smaller inhibitors as potential biological probes and ultimately, as therapeutic agents.

Biological Studies on TIMPs

Most studies to date have assessed the role and regulation of TIMP-1 in resorbing systems and less information on TIMP-2 is as yet available. Many connective tissue cells in culture synthesise TIMP-1 constitutively (Hembry et al., 1985), but levels of both protein and specific mRNA are elevated by a number of factors, including the cytokines, interleukin-1 α and β, tumor necrosis factor α, transforming growth factor β and basic fibroblast growth factor (Murphy et al., 1985; Edwards et al., 1987). Retinoids also stimulate TIMP biosynthesis (Clarke et al., 1987). Preliminary studies in our laboratory have shown that these effectors similarly modulate TIMP-2 production in fibroblasts. A major problem in assessing TIMP production by the use of activity assays has been the potential for interference by active MMPs. In particular, agents that modulate MMP production and activation can have effects on the levels of TIMP detectable in culture media e.g. corticosteroids inhibit MMP production by connective tissue cells giving an apparent elevation in TIMP production (McGuire-Goldring et al., 1983). Recently efforts have been made to overcome these problems, which equally well apply to MMP assays in the presence of TIMP (Murphy et al., 1989; Lefebvre & Vaes, 1989; Dean et al., 1989). The advent of immunoassays that distinguish TIMP in a free or complexed form should facilitate such studies (Cooksley et al., 1990).

The role of TIMPs may be to tightly regulate MMP activity at both the level of rate of proenzyme activation and subsequent substrate degradation. As with many other proteinase : inhibitor systems, activity may only be expressed at specific locations where inhibitor concentrations are reduced relative to that of MMPs. A number of cell model systems have been used to define the important role that TIMP can play in controlling matrix degradation, including normal connective tissue cells on collagen films (Gavrilovic et al., 1985) and tumor cells on amnion membranes (Thorgeirsson et al., 1982; Mignatti et al., 1986). TIMP has also been shown to effect a significant inhibition of metastatic lung colonisation by B16-F10 murine melanoma cells (Schultz et al., 1988). A number of studies of connective tissues have indicated that changes in TIMP-1 production by connective tissue cells are specifically associated with resorptive events. Both collagenase and TIMP could be immunolocalised in hypertrophic scar tissue undergoing active remodelling, but were not found in quiescent tissue (Hembry & Ehrlich, 1986). Similarly, very localised areas of remodelling in the fibrous joints of rabbit cranial sutures in response to mechanical force, are associated with regions of both collagenase and TIMP antigens (Green et al., 1990). In a colonic anastomoses model of wound healing in rabbits collagenase production was very specifically limited to the cut edges of the wound within 12h of resection. By 24h, TIMP was also detectable in the same region. New connective tissue sealing the serosal surface of the anastomosis also contained TIMP-secreting cells (Chowcat et al., 1988).

TIMP is likely to play an important role with respect to the control of tumour MMP activity, since it has been shown that there is a marked decrease in its production by malignant as compared with benign tumours (Halaka et al., 1983; Hicks et al., 1984). Recent experiments by Khokha et al., (1989) showed that antisense RNA induced a reduction in murine TIMP levels and conferred oncogenicity on Swiss 3T3 cells. MMPs and TIMP interactions may be regulatory steps in angiogenesis, a key step in the growth of large tumours. In a model system in which collagenase and gelatinase have been showed to be active, TIMP prevented the invasion of bovine capillary endothelial cells (stimulated with bFGF) into human amnion basement membrane (Mignatti et al., 1989). TIMP has also been shown to inhibit the metastatic potential of a highly metastatic rat embryo cell line, transfected by c-Ha-ras1 in order to induce secretion of gelatinases (Alvarez et al., 1990): large doses of TIMP injected intraperitoneally into nude mice prevented the metastasis to the lung of cells injected intravenously into the animals.

Evidence that tissue destruction in disease processes might result from an inbalance of MMPs over TIMPs is steadily accumulating. A reduction in TIMP synthesis relative to MMPs has been demonstrated by synovial explants from a rabbit model arthritis (Cambray et al., 1981) and from human rheumatoid synovium in culture (McGuire et al., 1981). In recent work, Dean et al., (1989) have found that extracts from osteoarthritic cartilage have considerably elevated levels of MMPs and only moderately increased levels of TIMP. High levels of TIMP-MMP complexes have been found in the synovial fluid of patients with septic arthritis (Cawston et al., 1990), with active MMPs present, but no free proteinase inhibitory activity. Using a collagen induced arthritis model Carmichael et al., (1989) have shown that systemic administration of recombinant TIMP can suppress the pathology.

Conclusion

The role of TIMPs in the regulation of MMP action during matrix turnover has been conclusively demonstrated in cell and animal model systems and initial data are becoming available concerning its inadequate production during degradative diseases. Besides developing these observations it will be important to observe the effect of enhancing TIMP levels *in vivo*. Our molecular understanding of the TIMPs is at a very early stage, but current work in this area will facilitate the development of specific low molecular weight inhibitors as potential therapeutic agents.

Acknowledgements

G.M. is supported by the Arthritis & Rheumatism Council, U.K. I am indebted to all my colleagues at Strangeways and at Celltech Limited, Slough, U.K. for their enthusiastic collaboration.

Referencess

Alvarez, O. A., Carmichael, D. F. and DeClerck, Y. A. (1990). J. Natl. Cancer Inst. 82: 589–595.

Boone, T. C., Johnson, M. J., De Clerck, Y. A. and Langley, K. E. (1990). Proc. Natl. Acad. Sci. USA 87: 2800–2804.

Bunning, R. A. D., Murphy, G., Kumar, S., Phillips, P. and Reynolds, J. J. (1984). Eur. J. Biochem. 139: 75–80.
Cambray, G. J., Murphy, G., Page-Thomas, D. P. and Reynolds, J. J. (1981). I. Synovium. Rheumatol. Int. 1: 11–16.
Carmichael, D. F., Sommer, A., Thompson, R. C., Anderson, D. C., Smith, C. G., Welgus, H. G. and Stricklin, G. P. (1986). Proc. Natl. Acad. Sci. USA 83: 2407–2411.
Carmichael, D. F., Stricklin, G. P. and Stuart, J. M. (1989). Agents Actions 27: 378–379.
Cawston, T. E. (1986). (Barrett, A. J. and Salvesen, G., eds), pp. 589–610. Elsevier Science Publishers BV.
Cawston, T., McLaughlan, P., Coughlan, R., Kyle, V. and Hazleman, B. (1990). Biochim. Biophys. Acta 1033: 96–102.
Cawston, T. E. and Mercer, E. (1986). FEBS Lett. 209: 9–12.
Cawston, T. E., Murphy, G., Mercer, E., Galloway, W. A., Hazleman, B. L. and Reynolds, J. J. (1983). Biochem. J. 211: 313–318.
Chowcat, N. L., Savage, F. J., Hembry, R. M. and Boulos, P. B. (1988). Br. J. Surg. 75: 330–334.
Clark, S. D., Kobayashi, D. K. and Welgus, H. G. (1987). J. Clin. Invest. 80: 1280–1288.
Cooksley, S., Hipkiss, J. B., Tickle, S. P., Holmes-levers, E., Docherty, A. J. P., Murphy, G. and Lawson, A. D. G. (1990). Matrix (in press).
Coulombe, B. and Skup, D. (1988). J. Biol. Chem. 263: 1439–1443.
Dean, D. D., Martel-Pelletier, J., Pelletier, J. P., Howell, D. S. and Woessner, J. F. (1989). J. Clin. Invest. 84: 678–685.
Docherty, A. J. P., Lyons, A., Smith, B. J., Wright, E. M., Stephens, P. E., Harris, T. J. R., Murphy, G. and Reynolds, J. J. (1985). Nature 318: 66–69.
Edwards, D. R., Murphy, G., Reynolds, J. J., Whitham, S. E., Docherty, A. J. P., Angel, P. and Heath, J. K. (1987). EMBO J. 6: 1899–1904.
Edwards, D. R., Waterhouse, P., Holman, M. L. and Denhardt, D. T. (1986). Nucleic Acids Res. 14: 8863–8878.
Galloway, W. A., Murphy, G., Sandy, J. D., Gavrilovic, J., Cawston, T. E. and Reynolds, J. J. (1983). Biochem. J. 209: 741–752.
Gavrilovic, J., Reynolds, J. J. and Murphy, G. (1985). Cell Biol. Int. Rep. 9: 1097–1107.
Green, D. D., Hembry, R. M., Atkinson, S. J., Reynolds, J. J. and Meikle, M. C. (1990). Am. J. Orthod. Dentofac. Orthop. 97: 281–288.
Halaka, A. N., Bunning, R. A. D., Bird, C. C., Gibson, M. and Reynolds, J. J. (1983). J. Neurosurg. 59: 461–466.
Hembry, R. M. and Ehrlich, H. P. (1986). Br. J. Dermatol. 115: 409–420.
Hembry, R. M., Murphy, G. and Reynolds, J. J. (1985). J. Cell Sci. 73: 105–119.
Hicks, N. J., Ward, R. V. and Reynolds, J. J. (1984). Int. J. Cancer 33: 835–844.
Horowitz, S., Dafni, N., Shapiro, D. L., Holm, B. A., Notter, R. H. and Quible, D. J. (1989). J. Biol. Chem. 264: 7092–7095.
Lefebvre, V. and Vaes, G. (1989). Biochim. Biophys. Acta 992: 355–361.

McGuire, M. B., Murphy, G., Reynolds, J. J. and Russell, R. G. G. (1981). Clin. Sci. 61: 703–710.

McGuire-Golddring, M. K. B., Murphy, G., Gowen, M., Meats, J. E., Ebsworth, N. M., Poll, C., Reynolds, J. J. and Russell, R. G. G. (1983). Biochim. Biophys. Acta 763: 129–139.

Mignatti, P., Robbins, E. and Rifkin, D. B. (1986). Cell 47: 487–498.

Mignatti, P., Tsuboi, R., Robbins, E. and Rifkin, D. B. (1989). J. Cell Biol. 108: 671–682.

Murphy, G., Koklitis, P. and Carne, A. F. (1989). Biochem. J. 261: 1031–1034.

Murphy, G., Reynolds, J. J. and Werb, Z. (1985). J. Biol. Chem. 260: 3079–3083.

Murray, J. B., Allison, K., Sudhalter, J. and Langer, R. (1986). J. Biol. Chem. 261: 4154–4159.

Schultz, R. M., Silberman, S., Persky, B., Bajkowski, A. S. and Carmichael, D. F. (1988). Cancer Res. 48: 5539–5545.

Stetler-Stevenson, W. G., Krutzsch, H. C. and Liotta, L. A. (1989). J. Biol. Chem. 264: 17374–17378.

Thorgeirsson, U. P., Kiotta, L. S., Kalebic, T., Margulies, I. M., Thomas, K., Rios-Candelore, M. and Russo, R. G. (1982). J. Natl. Cancer Inst. 69: 1049–1054.

Welgus, H. G., Jeffrey, J. J., Eisen, A. Z., Roswit, W. T. and Stricklin, G. P. (1985). Collagen Rel. Res. 5: 167–179.

Wilhelm, S. M., Collier, J. E., Marmer, B. L., Eisen, A. Z., Grant, G. A. and Goldberg, G. I. (1989). J. Biol. Chem. 264: 17213–17221.

Williamson, R. A., Marston, F. A. O., Angal, S., Koklitis, P., Panico, M., Morris, H. R., Carne, A. F., Smith, B. J., Harris, T. J. R. and Freedman, R. B. (1990). Biochem. J. 268: 267–274.

AAS 35
Progress in Inflammation
Research and Therapy

Probing the Role of Interleukin-1β Convertase in Interleukin-1β Secretion

A. D. Howard, N. Chartrain†, G. F. Ding*, M. J. Kostura*, G. Limjuco*, J. A. Schmidt*, M. J. Tocci†*

*The Department of Biochemical and Molecular Pathology and †The Department of Molecular Immunology, Merck Sharp and Dohme Research Laboratories, P.O. Box 2000 Rahway, NJ 07065, USA

Summary

Interleukin-1β must be processed from its precursor form of 31.5 kDa to its mature form of 17 kDa in order to elaborate its wide array of bioactivities. The recent identification of a monocyte-specific endoprotease, termed interleukin-1β-converting enzyme (ICE), capable of generating authentic, bioactive 17 kDa IL-1β suggests that this protease may serve a specific role in the processing and subsequent secretion of IL-1β. To test this hypothesis, we describe initial attempts to establish a monocytic cell-based system to test if mutant preIL-1β molecules which are poor substrates for ICE *in vitro* will be processed and secreted by monocytic cells.

Interleukin-1β (IL-1β) is a soluble polypeptide cytokine produced primarily by activated monocytes (Schmidt and Tocci, 1990; Dinarello and Savage, 1989). Considerable attention has been focused on the structure and bioactivities of this molecule. Surprisingly little is known concerning the processing and secretion of active IL-1β. The available evidence suggests that the proteolytic maturation and release of active IL-1β occurs by a novel pathway. Molecular coloning of IL-1β cDNAs from several species, biosynthetic studies in cultured cells and protein sequence analysis indicate that IL-1β is initially synthesized as a 31.5 kDa precursor (preIL-1β) devoid of biological activity which must be proteolytically cleaved to a 17.5 kDa mature form in order to acquire bioactivity (March et al., 1985; Mosley et al., 1987a; Mosley et al., 1987b; Hazuda et al.,

1989; Hazuda et al., 1985; Auron et al., 1984; Gray et al., 1986; Maliszewski et al., 1988; Mori et al., 1988). If this cleavage is due to a single endoproteolytic event, then it must occur between Asp-116 and Ala-117 since Ala-117 represents the authentic amino terminus of 17.5 kDa IL-1β (Cameron, 1986; Auron et al., 1987). Until recently, specific hydrolysis between an Asp-Ala sequence had not been described for a eukaryotic protease. Two independent studies have identified a monocyte-specific endoprotease, termed Interleukin-1β-Converting-Enzyme (ICE), which is capable of generating authentic, bioactive 17.5 kDa IL-1β by virtue of specific cleavage between Asp-116 and Ala 117 *in vitro* (Kostura et al., 1989; Black et al., 1989). Further work delineating the substrate specificity of ICE utilizing synthetic peptides (Sleath et al., 1990) or macromolecular substrates (Howard et al. 1990) has demonstrated that maintenance of Asp-116 is necessary for efficient catalysis, and Asp-Ala linkages must be in a proper, as yet undefined context, for cleavage by ICE.

In this report, we describe an approach to determine if ICE is involved in the processing and secretion of IL-1β in the living cell. We also review the distinctions and similarities between the two established processing and secretory pathways and compare them to what is known concerning the secretion of IL-1β.

Materials and Methods

Promonocytic U-937 cells were obtained from ATCC (Rockville, MD) and cultured in RPMI 1640 with 10% fetal bovine serum. The full-length cDNA encoding wild type or Ala-116 mutant precursor (Kostura et al., 1989) was placed under the control of the metallothionein II-A promoter. Transient transfections were carried out by liposome-mediated fusion using the lipofectin reagent with conditions supplied by the manufacturer (BRL/Gibco, Gaithesberg, MD). Expression of the transfected preIL-1β gene was induced 24 hours post transfection with PMA (30 ng/ml) and LPS (20 ng/ml). Transfectants were then metabolically radiolabeled with ^{35}S-methionine (1000 Ci/mmol, 125 uC/ml) and, after an additional 24 hours, cell lysates and culture supernatants were subjected to immunoprecipitation with anti-IL-1β antibodies followed by SDS-PAGE and fluorography.

Results and Discussion

The strategy we have adopted to define an *in vivo* role for ICE involves determining if preIL-1β cleavage site mutants which are refractory to cleavage *in vitro* would also not be cleaved *in vivo*. Since processing of preIL-1β is most likely obligatory for mature IL-1β secretion, prevention of *in vivo* processing of preIL-1β would be expected to block the secretion of these IL-1β molecules from the cell. The expression of mutant and wild type precursors in monocytic cell lines was carried out by transient transfection of their corresponding cDNA by liposome-mediated fusion. Promonocytic U-937 cells were chosen as the initial transfection host since they are readily transfectable unlike many monocytic cell lines. In addition, U-937 cells do not appear to contain ICE activity and synthesize small amounts of endogenous preIL-1β which is not secreted (Kostura and Howard, 1990). Following transfection, specific immunoprecipitates of metabolically radiolabeled cells show significant expression of preIL-1β over background levels (Fig. 1). PreIL-1β was only found intracellularly; no processed forms were found in cell culture supernatants. Expression was dependant on the post-transfection stimulation of the cells with PMA and LPS and was not due to the activation of the endogenous IL-1β gene since parallel transfections conducted with a cDNA containing preIL-1β in the reverse orientation or an irrelevant cDNA resulted in the synthesis of negligible amounts of preIL-1β. The most likely explanation for the finding that stimulation of the cells was a prerequisite for expression rests in the inducible nature of the metallothionein promoter (Karin et al., 1987) which drives expression of the transfected preIL-1β cDNA. These results demonstrate that expression of abundant amounts of preIL-1β in a monocytic cell line lacking ICE results in accumulation of intracellular precursor with no secretion of processed forms and extends similar findings observed in fibroblasts (Fuhlbrigge et al., 1988; Young et al., 1988) Similar experiments are in progress in the monocytic cell line, THP.1, the only cultured cell line reported to date which contains ICE activity and is capable of processing and secreting mature IL-1β (Matsushima et al., 1985; Kostura et al., 1989; Black et al., 1989).

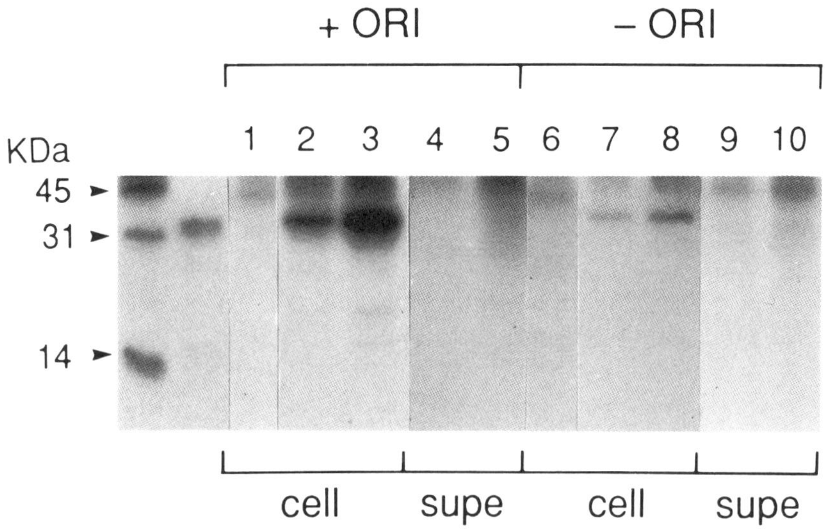

Figure 1. Transient expression of preIL-1β by U-937 cells. U-937 cells were transfected and analyzed as described in *Materials and Methods*. Lanes 1–5, positive orientation wild type preIL-1β transfectants; lanes 6–10, negative orientation wild type preIL-1β transfectants. Treatments: lanes 1, 6 = no treatment; 2, 4, 7, 9 = PMA alone; 3, 5, 8, 10 = PMA + LPS. Cell lysates and culture supernatents were immunoprecipitated with specific anti-IL-1β antisera. As a size standard, 31 kDa preIL-1β is shown in the second lane from the left.

In recent years, a great deal of progress has been made in the elucidation of the cellular mechanisms responsible for the biosynthesis, processing and secretion of peptide hormones. The general scheme that has emerged involves removal of a hydrophobic signal sequence as the nascent polypeptide enters the lumen of the endoplasmic reticulum followed by proteolytic processing at paired basic residues of a larger, typically inactive precursor (Fisher and Scheller, 1988) Liberation of the active peptide from the cell can occur as fast as it is synthesized (constitutive secretion) or can be stored and concentrated in secretory vesicles and released upon treatment with an appropriate secreatogue (regulated secretion) (Kelly, 1985). This pathway is exemplified in the cleavage of yeast alpha-mating factor by KEX 2 endoprotease (Fuller et al., 1988). It is apparent, however, that the above paradigm for processing and secretion is not applicable for all secreted peptides. The prime examples of divergent behaviour from the classical pathway are typified by yeast a-mating factor and bacterial hemolysin A (Fuller et al., 1988; McGrath and Varshavsky, 1989; Powers et al., 1986; Clark and Sprague, 1989; Koronakis et al., 1989). In the case of a-factor, this protein lacks a signal sequence (N-terminal or internal) necessary for the transloca-tion of the nascent protein across the ER membrane, appears to be synthesized on cytoplasmic ribosomes rather than membrane-bound ribosomes, and therefore lack N-linked carbohydrate. In addition, a-factor undergoes a strikingly unique set of covalent modifications during its maturation to its mature form. These include acylation with fatty acids or isoprenoids and proteolytic processing at atypical sites. A variety of genetic and functional criteria have begun to delineate the existence of other genes and gene products intimately involved in the processing and secretion of both a-mating factor and hemolysis A. These sequences encode transport/translocation proteins which are homologs of the mammalian multi-drug resis-tance P-glycoprotein (for a-factor, the STE 6 gene product) or maturation enzymes (for a-factor the RAM 1 gene product). The above observations suggest the existence of an alternative secretory mechanism involving at least two basic steps: modification of the protein with lipid which engenders a membrane seeking character, and interaction of the modified protein with an integral membrane translocation factor and transport out of the cell. The above obser-vations imply that the alternative secretory pathway is conserved evolutionarily.

Several lines of evidence point to a unique pathway of IL-1β processing and secretion whcih may resemble the alternative path-way discussed above. All IL-1β sequences characterized lack a hydrophobic signal motif (Auron et al, 1984; March et al., 1985; Gray et al., 1986; Maliszewski et al., 1988; Mori et al., 1988). A recent study has shown that preIL-1β but not the mature form appears to be modified by fatty acid (Bursten et al., 1988). Precursor IL-1β, when expressed *in vitro*, is incapable of translocation across competent microsomal membranes (Limjuco and Kostura, 1990; Hogquist and Chaplin, 1990). Light and electron microscopic studies immunolocalize IL-1β to the cytoplasm and fail to demonstrate IL-1β in the organelles that are involved in classical secretion

(Bayne et al., 1986; Singer et al., 1988). Taken together, the above observations infer a unique secretory pathway for IL-1β.

References

Auron, P. E., Rossenwasser, L. J., Mucci, S. F., Rich, A., Wolff, S. M. and Dinarello, C. M. (1984). Nucleotide sequence of human monocyte interleukin-1 precursor cDNA. Proc. Natl. Acad. Sci. USA 81: 7907.

Bayne, E. K., Rupp, E., Limjuco, G., Chin, J. and Schmidt, J. A. (1986). Immunocytochemical detection of interleukin-1 within stimulated human monocytes. J. Exp. Med. 163: 1267.

Black, R. A., Kronheim, S. R. and Sleath, P. R. (1989). Activation of interleukin-1β by a co-induced protease. FEBS Lett. 247: 386.

Bursten, S. L., Locksley, R. M., Ryan, J. L. and Lovett, D. H. (1988). Acylation of monocyte and glomerular mesangial cell proteins – myristyl acylation of the interleukin-1 precursors. J. Clin. Invest. 82: 1479.

Cameron, P. M., Limjuco, G. A., Chin, J., Silberstein, L. and Schmidt, J. A. (1986). Purification to homogeneity and amino acid sequence analysis of two anionic species of human interleukin-1. J. Exp. Med. 164: 237.

Clark, K. L. and Sprague, G. F. (1989). Yeast pheromone response pathway: characterization of a suppressor that restores mating to receptorless mutants. Mol. Cell. Biol. 9: 2682.

Dinarello, C. A. and Savage, N. (1989). Interleukin-1 and it's receptor. Critical Rev. in Immunol. 9: 1.

Dixon, M. and Webb, E. C. (1979). Enzyme Specificity In Enzymes, Academic Press, New York, NY, p. 231.

Fuhlbrigge, R. C., Fine, S. M., Unanue, E. R. and Chaplin, D. D. (1988). Expression of membrane interleukin-1 by fibroblasts transfected with murine prointerleukin-1α cDNA. Proc. Natl. Acad. Sci. USA 85: 5649.

Gray, P. W., Glaister, D., Chen, E., Goeddel, D. V. and Pennica, D. (1986). Two interleukin-1 genes in the mouse: cloning and expression of the cDNA for murine interleukin-1β. J. Immunol. 137: 3644.

Hazuda, D., Webb, R. L., Simon, P. and Young, P. (1989). Purification and characterization of human recombinant precursor interleukin-1β. J. Biol. Chem. 264: 16896.

Hazuda, D., Lee, J. C. and Young, P. (1988). The kinetics of interleukin-1 secretion from activated monocytes. J. Biol. Chem. 263: 8473.

Hogquist, K. and Chaplin, D. D. (1990). Unpublished observations.

Howard, A. D, Kostura, M. J., Ding, G., Limjuco, G., Cameron, P., Hogquist, K., Chaplin, D. D., Schmidt, J. A. and Tocci, M. J. (1990). Manuscript submitted.

Karin, M., Haslinger, A., Heguy, A., Dietlin, T. and Cooke, T. (1987). Metal-reponsive elements act as positive regulators of human metallothionein enhancer activity. Mol. Cell. Biol. 7: 606.

Koronakis, U., Koronakis, E. and Hughes, C. (1989). Isolation and analysis of the C-terminal signal directing export of Escherichia coli hemolysin protein across bacterial membranes. EMBO J. 8: 595.

Kostura, M. J., Tocci, M. J., Limjuco, G., Chin, J., Cameron, P., Hillman, A., Chartrain, N. and Schmidt, J. A. (1989). Identification of a monocyte specific interleukin-1 convertase activity. Proc. Natl. Acad. Sci. USA 86: 5227.

Kostura, M. J. and Howard, A. D. (1990). Unpublished observations.

Limjuco, G. and Kostura, M. J. (1990). Unpublished observations.

Maliszewski, C. R., Baker, P. E., Schoenborn, M. A., Davis, B. S., Cosman, D., Killis, S. and Cerretti, D. P. (1988). Cloning and expression of bovine interleukin-1α and interleukin-1β complementary DNAs. Mol. Immunol. 25: 429.

March, C. J., Mosley, B., Larsen, A., Cerretti, D. P., Braedt, G., Price, V., Gillis, S., Henney, C., Kronheim, S. R., Grabstein, K., Conlon, P. J., Hopp T. P. and Cosman, D. (1985). Cloning, sequence and expression of two distinct human interleukin-1 cDNAs. Nature 315: 641.

Matsushima, K., Copeland, T. D., Onozaki, K. and Oppenheim, J. J. (1985). Purification and bochemical characterization of two distinct human interleukins-1 from the myeloblastic THP-1 cell line. J. Immunol. 135: 1132.

McGrath, J. P. and Varshavsky, A. (1989). The yeast STE6 gene encodes a homologue of the mammalian multidrug resistance P-glycoprotein. Nature 340: 400.

Mori S., Goto, K., Ohkawara, S., Maeda, S., Shimada, K. and Yoshinaga, M. (1988). Cloning and sequence analysis of a cDNA for lymphocyte proliferation protentiating factor of rabbit polymorphonuclear leukocytes: identification as rabbit interleukin-1β. Biochem. Biophys. Res. Commun. 150: 1237.32.

Mosley, B., Urdal, D. L., Prickett, K. S., Larsen, A., Cosman, D., Conlon, P. J., Gillis, S. and Dower, S. K. (1987a). The interleukin-1 receptor binds the interleukin-1α precursor but not the interleukin-1β precursor. J. Biol. Chem. 262: 2941.

Mosley, B., Dower, S., Gillis, S. and Cosman, D. (1987b). Determination of the minimum polypeptide lengths of the functionally active sites of human interleukins-1α and β. Proc. Natl. Acad. Sci. USA. 84: 4572.

Powers, S., et al. (1986). RAM, a gene of yeast required for a functional modification of RAS proteins and for production of mating pheromone a-factor. Cell 47: 413.

Schmidt, J. A. and Tocci, M. J. (1990). Interleukin-1. In The Handbook of Experimental Pharmacology, Vol. 95, I, Peptide Growth Factors and their Receptors, M. Sporn and A. Roberts, editors. Springer Verlag, 473–521.

Singer, I., Scott, S., Hall, G. L., Limjuco, G., Chin, J. and Schmidt, J. A. (1988). Interleukin-1β is localized in the cytoplasmic ground substance but is largely absent from the golgi apparatus and plasma membrane of stimulated human monocytes. J. Exp. Med. 167: 389.

Sleath, P. R., Hendrickson, R. C., Kronheim, S. R., March C. J. and Black, R. A. (1990). Substrate specificity of the protease that processes human interleukin-1β. J. Biol. Chem. 265: 14526.

Young, P. R., Hazuda, D. H. and Simon, P. (1988). Human interleukin-1β is not secreted from hamster fibroblasts when expressed constitutively from a transfected cDNA. J. Cell. Biol. 107: 447.

AAS 35
Progress in Inflammation
and Research and Therapy

The Proteolytic Activation of Interleukin-1β

*R. Black, S. Kronheim, P. Sleath, T. Greenstreet, G. Duke Virca, C. March and T. Kupper**

Department of Protein Chemistry, Immunex Corp., 51 University St., Seattle, WA 98101, USA and *Departments of Medicine (Dermatology) and Pathology, Washington University School of Medicine, St. Louis, MO 63110, USA

Summary

Interleukin-1β (IL-1β) is released from an inactive precursor by a proteolytic cleavage. A monocytic protease has been identified that appears to be involved in the physiological activation of this cytokine. Two situations have been found in which precursor IL-1β exists without the monocytic processing enzyme, and in these cases other proteases, such as neutrophil elastase, cathepsin G and cathepsin L, may be involved in generating the active cytokine.

Mature IL-1β consists of the C-terminal 153 amino acids of an inactive 269-amino-acid precursor (March et al., 1985). The N-terminal amino acid of the mature cytokine, alanine-117 of the precursor, is not preceded by a typical sequence for processing, such as a pair of basic residues. However, the aspartate preceding the mature N-terminus is strictly conserved across species (Cannon et al., 1989), suggesting the possibility of an unusual, aspartate-specific processing enzyme. We and others have in fact found such an enzyme in monocytes, the primary source of IL-1β (Black et al., 1989b; Kostura et al., 1989). This paper reviews the evidence that proteolysis is required for the generation of active IL-1β and that the aspartate-specific protease is involved in the physiological activation of this cytokine. We also describe two situations in which precursor IL-1β is found without this protease, and we discuss other enzymes which may be involved in processing in these cases.

Material and Methods

Recombinant pro-IL-1β and mature IL-1β were prepared as previously described (Black et al., 1988). Neutrophil elastase and cathepsin G were obtained from Elastin Products. Recombinant cathepsin L (in the zymogen form) was expressed in yeast, purified from the yeast culture medium, and acid-activated prior to use.

The digestion of pro-IL-1β and analysis of the digests by Western blot were carried out as previously described (Black et al., 1988), except that the buffer for the digestion with cathepsin L was 100 mM sodium acetate, 10 mM acetic acid, 1 mM EDTA, 4 mM dithiothreitol (pH 5.5).

Results and Discussion

The first indication that pro-IL-1β is inactive came from attempts to clone IL-1 using reticulocyte lysates (March et al., 1985). Biological activity due to IL-1α could be detected in reticulocyte lysate translations of mRNA from monocytes, but activity due to IL-1β was not found in this system. Mosley and Dower subsequently showed that only the 31 kilodalton precursor of IL-1β is made by reticulocyte lysates supplied with the mRNA encoding this protein, and that the precursor does not bind to the IL-1 receptor (Mosley et al., 1987).

To pursue how the initial translation product is activated, we expressed the precursor in *E. coli*, partially purified it, and tested whether proteolytic cleavage alone is sufficient to produce biologically active IL-1β. We found that digestion with chymotrypsin generated an 18 kilodalton form of IL-1β (the mature cytokine is 17.5 kilodaltons) and concomitantly increased activity about 500-fold (Black et al., 1988).

The monocytic cell line THP-1 was used as a potential source of the physiologically relevant processing enzyme. We found that a lysate of these cells does produce the mature cytokine from the recombinant precursor, and that this processing activity was due to a single, unusual protease (Black et al., 1989b). This protease was found to have an absolute requirement for aspartate in the P1 position of its substrates (Sleath et al., 1990): while it cleaved a synthetic substrate representing residues 112–121 of the precursor, replacing the residue corresponding to Asp-116 with Glu, Asn or D-Asp prevented cleavage.

This monocytic processing enzyme is thus specific for the one amino acid at the cleavage site, aspartate, that is conserved across species, and we have shown by pulse-chase analysis that monocytes in fact generate mature IL-1β by an endoproteolytic cleavage at the aspartate-alanine bond of the precursor (Black et al., 1990). A further line of evidence pointing to a physiological role for this protease is that its expression correlates with that of IL-1β in stimulated THP-1 cells (Black et al., 1989b).

Two situations have been found, however, in which the precursor exists in the absence of this protease. Stimulated human monocytes secrete large amounts of pro-IL-1β (Hazuda et al., 1988), and we have found that even THP-1 cells, which contain a high level of processing activity, actually secrete more precursor than mature IL-1β. We have never observed any processing of this extracellular material. This finding is consistent with the observation that all the aspartate-specific monocytic protease is cell-associated, but it raises the possibility that *in vivo* other proteases may act on the released precursor.

A second case where other proteases may be involved is the human keratinocyte. All the IL-1 activity in keratinocyte lysates is due to IL-1α, but we have found that these cells contain substantial amounts of precursor IL-1β (Mizutani et al., submitted). ELISA assays indicated that there is about as much IL-1β as there is IL-1α in keratinocyte lysates, and Western plot analysis indicated that the lysates contain a protein of about 31 kilodaltons that reacts with antibodies to IL-1β. To confirm that this protein is pro-IL-1β, we digested the lysate with chymotrypsin. This treatment converted the 31 kilodalton protein to an 18 kilodalton form, as expected if it were IL-1β, and the digestion increased the IL-1 activity of the material. Thus keratinocytes do contain precursor IL-1β.

The precursor found without the aspartate-specific processing enzyme could serve some non-cytokine function, or it could be processed, *in vivo*, by some other protease. To test whether proteases known to be associated with inflammation could play a processing role, we incubated recombinant pro-IL-1β with neutrophil elastase and cathepsin G, two enzymes released by neutrophils, and with

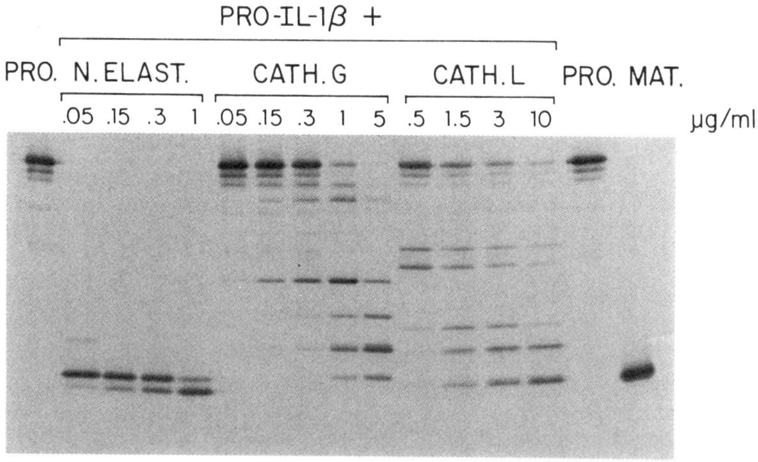

Figure 1. Digestion of pro-IL-1β by proteases associated with inflammation. The precursor was incubated with the indicated concentrations of each protease (except that the concentrations of elastase were 1000-fold greater than indicated) for 30 min. at 37°C., and the digests were then analyzed by Western blot.

cathepsin L, which is secreted by macrophages. As shown in Figure 1, all three proteases do generate mature or near-mature forms of IL-1β from the precursor. (Similar data with elastase and cathepsin G have also been reported by others (Hazuda et al., 1990).)

We have also found a novel protease in the medium of PHA-stimulated peripheral blood cells that cleaves the precursor on the amino-terminal side of aspartate-116, rather than on the carboxy side (Black et al., 1989a).

It remains uncertain whether any proteases other than the monocytic, aspartate-specific enzyme are actually involved in IL-1β processing *in vivo*. We do not know whether either monocytes or keratinocytes ever release the precursor *in vivo*, nor do we know whether the other proteases described would efficiently process low concentrations of the precursor. Finally, it is possible that even if some precursor is released physiologically and these proteases are capable of processing it, mature IL-1β produced by the monocytic enzyme we have identified is required to induce the secretion of these proteases. Experiments with specific inhibitors of the monocytic processing enzyme will be required to determine if it is a useful target for reducing the inflammatory damage caused by IL-1β.

References

Black, R. A., Kronheim, S. R., Cantrell, M., Deeley, M. C., March, C. J., Prickett, K. S., Wignall, J., Conlon, P. J., Cosman, D., Hopp, T. P. and Mochizuki, D. Y. (1988). J. Biol. Chem. 263: 9437–9442.

Black, R. A., Kronheim, S. R., Merriam, J. E., March, C. J. and Hopp, T. P. (1989a). J. Biol. Chem. 264: 5323–5326.

Black, R. A., Kronheim, S. R. and Sleath, P. R. (1989b). FEBS Lett. 247: 386–390.

Black, R. A., Kronheim, S. R., Sleath, P. R., Greenstreet, T. A., Van Ness, K. P., Glackin, P. J., Griffin, A., Hendrickson, R. C., Merriam, M. A. and March, C. J. (1990). In: Molecular and Cellular Biology of Cytokines (J. J. Oppenheim, M. C. Powanda, M. J. Kluger and C. A. Dinarello, Eds). Wiley-Liss, New York. pp. 69–74.

Cannon, J. G., Clark, B. D., Wingfield, P., Schmeissner, U., Losberger, C., Dinarello, C. A. and Shaw, A. R. (1989). J. Immunol. 142: 2299–2306.

Hazuda, D. J., Lee, J. C. and Young, P. R. (1988). J. Biol. Chem. 263: 8473–8479.

Hazuda, D. J., Strickler, J., Keuppers, F., Simon, P. L. and Young, P. R. (1990). J. Biol. Chem. 265: 6318–6322.

Kostura, M. J., Tocci, M. J., Limjuco, G., Chin, J., Cameron, P., Hillman, A. G., Chartrain, N. A. and Schmidt, J. A. (1989). Proc. Natl. Acad. Sci. U.S.A. 86: 5227–5231.

March, C. J., Mosley, B., Larsen, A., Cerretti, D. P., Braedt, G., Price, V., Gillis, S., Henney, C. S., Kronheim, S. R., Grabstein, K., Conlon, P. J., Hopp, T. P. and Cosman, D. (1985). Nature. 316: 641–647.

Mizutani, H., Black, R. A. and Kupper, T. S. J. Clin. Invest. (submitted).

Mosley, B., Urdal, D. L., Prickett, K. S., Larsen, A., Cosman, D., Conlon, P. J., Gillis, S. and Dower, S. K. (1987). J. Biol. Chem. 262: 2941–2944.

Sleath, P. R., Hendrickson, R. C., Kronheim, S. R., March, C. J. and Black, R. A. (1990). J. Biol. Chem. 265: 14526–14528.

Clinical Aspects

Progress in Inflammation
Research and Therapy

NSAID Association with Gastrointestinal Bleeding and Peptic Ulcer

B. I. Hirschowitz and A. Lanas

Division of Gastroenterology, University of Alabama at Birmingham, Birmingham, AL 35294, USA

Summary

This paper reviews recent data describing the increased risk of bleeding and peptic ulcer with NSAID use in arthritis and non-arthritis populations. We briefly report personal studies on both aspects. By objective testing in 66 GI bleeders the use of NSAIDs, especially ASA, was more strongly associated with GI bleeding from both ulcer and non-ulcer sources, including colonic, than previously reported (82% vs. 21% in controls). ASA abuse, often surreptitious, may account for many, if not most, treatment-resistant peptic ulcers. We report 29 such patients. Adverse effects of NSAID use add considerably to economic cost, excess morbidity and mortality, especially in the elderly. Bleeding and peptic ulcer are separate risks of NSAID use. This conclusion carries major implications for prophylaxis strategies.

There is a growing awareness that NSAID damage to the human GI tract produces a significant morbidity and excess mortality in patients dependent upon these drugs. In the US in 1986 70,000,000 prescriptions for NSAIDs were dispensed. Add to that the manufacture of 12,000 tons of aspirin (ASA) or the equivalent of 40 billion ASA doses sold under scores of trade names and formulations, plus other nonprescription (OTC) NSAIDs, thus exposing a very large, medically unsupervised population to risk of serious GI lesions. Such risk may be estimated from the 21–25% incidence of side effects of NSAIDs in the UK and USA (Langman, 1988; Ehsanullah et al. 1988; Butt et al., 1988), representing one-fourth of all reported drug side effects (Langman, 1988). These add 45% to the already high medical cost of arthritis (Bloom, 1988). Such side effects are all the more dangerous because 40% of NSAIDs users are over 60 years old (Baum et al., 1985).

GI side effects of NSAIDs can be divided into those causing symptoms (nausea, anorexia, dyspepsia, heartburn, pain), those causing new or exacerbating old gastric or duodenal ulcer and those causing life threatening complications such as bleeding or perforation and which can occur without warning. Depending on dose, the relative risk of peptic ulcer or bleeding is variously cited as 1.5 to 12 (Faulkner et al., 1988; Kurata and Abbey, 1990). Though the risk is relatively low, the large numbers of persons using these drugs translates into a substantial and growing number of major complications.

We will present data that show a much larger role for NSAIDs particularly ASA, in GI bleeding and in nonhealing of peptic ulcer.

Mucosal Damage

From a practical clinical point of view the degrees of mucosal damage should be graded into those that are and those that are not clinically significant or likely to be subject to life threatening complications (Barrier and Hirschowitz, 1989).

Endoscopically the degrees of damage visible to the naked eye are petechiae, seen commonly after acute ingestion of ASA or NSAIDs, most frequently in the antrum and becoming less prevalent after continued intake (Graham et al. 1988). This type of lesion (which we call Grade I) is the kind seen in normal volunteers used to study acute NSAIDs "gastropathy" (Graham and Smith, 1986; Ivey, 1986; Roth, 1988; Silen, 1988). They are trivial findings of no consequence except as possible markers of NSAID use. The next level (Grade II) is represented by small erosions (superficial ulcers that do not penetrate the muscularis mucosae) of the antrum which occur dose dependently in patients taking NSAIDs or ASA chronically (Faulkner et al., 1988). These do not progress to Grade III. They are clearly distinguishable from acute stress erosions. Stress ulcers which occur in the gastric body and fundus always have an element of vascular damage and are prone to bleed, while the ASA ulcers in the antrum seldom do. Grade III lesions are the classical chronic deep peptic ulcers penetrating the muscularis which may, and most often do, occur independently of NSAID use. Ten to 15% of regular NSAIDs users have chronic ulcers, and it is this population that is at risk for bleeding and perforation. For purposes of understanding NSAID lesions of the upper GI tract, Grade I and II lesions are considered to be not clinically dangerous (and may occur with or without symptoms) while Grade III lesions are potentially serious lesions, 20% of which are asymptomatic (Ehsanullah et al., 1988), including many that develop further complications.

Symptoms

Some combination of nausea, dyspepsia, anorexia, pain or heartbuen is reported in 20–25% of patients taking NSAIDs chronically (Ehsanullah et al., 1988) though extremes of incidence from 8 to 60% are reported (Semble and Wu, 1987; Coles et al., 1983; Caruso and Bianchi Porro, 1980). Symptoms are usually, though not always, dose related (Graham et al., 1988) and are not always associated with visible damage. In one study, 21% of the patients taking therapeutic doses of NSAIDs were symptomatic (Ehsanullah et al., 1988). Eighteen percent of the symptomatic patients had a normal endoscopy, and another 40% only minor lesions (Grade I or II) and 40% had Grade III lesions (chronic ulcer). In a number of instances patients with symptomatic ulcer take NSAID to relieve such symptoms. This is especially seen with AlkaSeltzer which combines antacid and ASA. Such use carries the risk of inducing bleeding. The masking of warning symptoms is more prevalent in the elderly who also are more prone to bleeding and perforation induced by NSAIDs (Skander and Ryan, 1988; Doherty et al., 1987).

Bleeding

Bleeding is a recognized complication of NSAID treatment. Occult bleeding is dose related (Graham and Smith, 1986) and by ^{51}Cr labelling can be documented in as many as 3 out of 4 chronic ASA users (Pierson et al., 1961; Lussier and LeBel, 1987) and may or may not be associated with visible mucosal lesions. The usual rate of loss of 2–3 ml/day is clinically insignificant compared to the normal loss of 1 ml/day (Graham and Smith, 1986). Some susceptible individuals may lose as much as or more than 10 ml/day which may cause anemia. Such a result may be hard to distinguish from anemia of chronic disease.

Compared to the above, massive acute GI bleeding should be considered to be a separate manifestation of NSAID complications (Faulkner et al., 1988: Bartle et al., 1986; Carson et al., 1987). Chronic ulcers are the ones most likely to bleed or perforate. The risk of bleeding is not well defined, but is probably much higher than in ulcer patients not taking NSAIDs. Bleeding and ulcer formation may be considered separate and additive risks. By history one in three upper GI bleeders studied in the UK (Faulkner et al., 1988) could be directly attributed to NSAIDs and one-third of those were due to ASA, giving a risk ratio over case controls of 1.5. The risk of bleeding from NSAIDs was estimated in the UK to be 1 per 20,000 months; in the US a retrospective study of 47,000 patients in Michigan and Minnesota (Carson et al., 1987) yielded a risk of 1.9 per 10,000 patient treatment months. Kurata and Abbey, 1990, studied prospectively for upper GI complications some 2500 non-ulcer cardiac patients taking 1 gram ASA daily for 4 years compared to 2500 controls. Upper GI bleeding requiring hospital admission occurred in 14 persons in the ASA users compared to 0 in controls for a rate of 1.2 per 10,000 months, a value similar to that of Carson et al., 1987.

Personal Studies

We have re-examined the association of NSAID intake and GI bleeding using methodology that provided objective evidence of current NSAID intake and have arrived at a much higher estimate than obtained from historical data. (Lanas et al., 1991). We studied prospectively GI bleeding patients and nonbleeding controls admitted to hospital. To establish an objective test of current NSAIDs use, we measured platelet cyclooxygenase activity by the production of thromboxane B2 from labelled arachidonic acid (Connor and Laposata, 1988).

In 66 bleeders, 48 patients had objective evidence of a current ASA use and another 6 had used other NSAIDs within 2 to 5 days of admission for bleeding for a total prevalence of 83%, significantly higher ($p < 0.001$) compared to 21% of 38 case controls who were matched for age and sex. This gives an odds ratio of 10.2 for an NSAID effect on GI bleeding. ASA accounted for 90% of the NSAID associated with bleeding. GI bleeding was further broken down according to source. Peptic ulcer was the source in 28 patients (14 DU, 14 GU); other upper GI lesions (Mallory Weiss, AV malformation, varices) accounted for another 17 of whom 65% had evidence of current NSAID use, for an odds ratio of NSAID use in ulcer vs. non-ulcer in upper GI bleeders of 4.5. What was surprising and even alarming was that 86% of 22 patients who bled from the colon had evidence of NSAID use. The odds ratio of lower GI vs. upper GI bleeding in NSAID users was 1.05 indicating no predilection for site. Severity of bleeding was not different between NSAID positive and negative bleeders. (Lanas et al., 1991).

The strong association of current NSAID use and GI bleeding from both ulcer and non-ulcer sources suggests that NSAIDs, especially ASA, may be a more pervasive and dangerous cause for GI bleeding of all types than has been previously recognized, and regardless of the reason for taking NSAIDS. The problem then should be redefined since the conventional view of the risk of NSAID therapy is perceived as NSAID --> ulcer --> bleeding. The risk can now be viewed as a direct one, NSAID (esp. ASA) --> bleeding, with chronic peptic ulcer, whether from NSAID or not, being only one of many risk factors. This view has important implications for prophylactic treatment strategies. Thus prostaglandins, even if they reduce the incidence of GU (Graham, 1989) would not prevent clinically significant bleeding from either DU or non-ulcer upper or lower GI bleeding. In fact, two of the present duodenal ulcer bleeders were taking misoprostil (Cytotec). If bleeding occurs more frequently from non-ulcer, including non-gastric, sources, the basis of calculating cost effectiveness of misoprostil prophylaxis (Edelson et al., 1990) may be drastically changed for the worse.

It is not known why only some people bleed upon the ingestion of ASA or other NSAIDs. Inactivation of platelets by ASA is irreversible and recovery requires replacement by generation of new platelets. Whether there are any additional effects on platelets or vessels in bleeders remains to be shown. It is also evident that bleeding carries a significantly higher risk for older patients who represent 40% of the NSAIDs users (Baum et al., 1985), and in whom almost all the deaths from ulcer complications occur (Armstrong and Blower, 1987; Griffin et al., 1988).

Chronic Ulcers

It is generally agreed that excessive use of aspirin may cause gastric ulcers (Piper et al., 1982). Between 15 and 20% of those taking 2.4 gm ASA per day have chronic gastric ulcers and twice that many have erosions (Grade II lesions). Graham and Smith (1986) calculated the relative risk of gastric ulcer >1.0 with 22 tablets per week, i.e. 1 gm/day, reaching 5.0 with 40 tablets/week. Kurata and Abbey (1990), however, in non-ulcer patients in a cardiac prophylaxis study using 1 gm ASA/day, report an adjusted relative risk for DU of 10.7 and of GU of 9.1 in patients with symptoms serious enough to be admitted to hospital. These figures probably represent an underestimate of the absolute incidence, since only those hospitalized for DU or GU were counted. The ARAMIS study of Fries et al. (1989) in treated arthritics reports a risk ratio of 6.45 for NSAIDs users for GI disease hospitalizations. Denis McCarthy (personal communication) has estimated from 6 NSAID and 2 ASA post-marketing studies the annual risk of developing a peptic ulcer as between 4 and 6%. It is thus clear that ASA use is as much related to excess risk of DU as for GU.

Non-healing Ulcer

A different but related association between NSAIDs and peptic ulcer is manifested by the prevention of healing. Perrault et al. (1988) reported 5 cases of treatment resistant ulcers due to surreptitious use of ASA. In 4 of the 5 patients surgery was followed by relapse of ulcer despite achlorhydria. We have found 29 such patients in 2 1/2 years in whom duodenal ($n = 11$), gastric ($n = 7$), marginal ($n = 4$) or esophageal ($n = 3$) ulceration alone or in various combinations was associated with persistent ASA use, discovered by the presence of salicylate in serum after at least 10 hours fast. Four of these patients (and 4 others not studied before surgery) who had surgery for intractable ulcer had recurrent (marginal) ulcers within one year with continuing evidence of ASA abuse. Seventy-six percent of the 29 patients denied use of ASA despite repeated demonstration of salicylate in serum. Over the course of observation all 29 patients were resistant to treatment with H2 antagonists, usually with added carafate. The majority who were so treated responded to (often repeated) courses of omeprazole in 4 to 8 weeks, relapsing on substitution with H2 antagonists. In controls with ulcers that healed normally, no salicylates were detected.

This population of surreptitious or inadvertent ASA users may well represent the majority of patients who fail conventional ulcer therapy and who do not have Zollinger-Ellison Syndrome. Serum salicylate and serum gastrin measurements should be included in the workup of all treatment resistant cases. Those abusing ASA should not be operated on except for surgical emergencies.

Recommendations for NSAID-Treated Patients

The development of symptoms or complications poses a serious dilemma for the patient whose treatment is dependent upon NSAID. Since complications are dose related, the lowest effective dose should be used. Yet 75 to 80% of patients taking NSAIDs are free of symptoms and only 5% of these are at risk of having an ulcer and a smaller percentage of bleeding. These patients do not require endoscopy.

The 20 to 25% of patients with GI symptoms that persist despite alteration of dose or frequency of medication should be investigated for upper GI lesions. In 40% of this group these lesions are significant (chronic GU or DU) and potentially hazardous. These patients should be treated with H2 antagonists, which if successful might be continued long-term. Such patients require follow-up to assure the physician of healing since unhealed ulcers remain a serious bleeding risk, even if asymptomatic. If this therapy does not heal the ulcer, omeprazole (Losec) may be effective within 4 to 8 weeks (Walan et al., 1989). However, long-term treatment with omeprazole is not yet approved or recommended for this indication. Symptoms with Grade II lesions should also be treated with H2 antagonists, but may not require treatment beyond that necessary to suppress symptoms. In either case if cotherapy is ineffective or required indefinitely, consideration should be given to use of arthritis medication other than NSAIDs.

There is no evidence to support the use of sucralfate, antacids or prostaglandins for treating gastric or duodenal ulcers due to NSAIDs (McCarthy, 1989).

Prophylaxis

Those patients who have a history of duodenal ulcer and who need NSAIDs should have cotreatment with H2 antagonists (Ehsanullah et al., 1988); those who had a gastric ulcer might be cotreated with misoprostol (Graham, 1989) though its efficacy remains to be proven in further studies. There is some difficulty in selecting rational prophylaxis for patients who have previously bled (see above). While all NSAIDs have been implicated in causing bleeding, most of the bleeding episodes were ASA related in our study. Thus at least ASA should be avoided in any patient with a history of ulcer or bleeding. It may be that reversible inhibitors of platelet cyclooxygenase activity such as ibuprofen may be better than the irreversible inhibitor ASA, but that remains to be specifically studied. General prescription of either H2 antagonists or of misoprostol does not make therapeutic or economic sense, since neither actually prevents bleeding other than possibly through selective but imperfect prevention of duodenal or gastric ulcer, respectively.

Much further prospective post-marketing data are required to determine relative risk of various NSAIDs. Further progress will be made when we determine whether the therapeutic and adverse effects of these drugs depend on the same or different mechanisms.

References

Armstrong, C. P. and Blower, A. L. (1987). Gut 28: 527–532.

Barrier, C. H. and Hirschowitz, B. I. (1989). Arthritis and Rheumatism 32: 926–932.

Barle, W. R., Gupta, A. K. and Lazor, J. (1986). Arch. Intern. Med. 146: 2365–2367.

Baum, C., Kennedy, D. L. and Forbes. M. B. (1985). Arthritis Rheum. 28: 686–692.
Bloom, B. S. (1988). Aliment. Pharmacol. Ther. 2S: 131–139.
Butt, J. H., Barthel, J. S. and Moore, R. A. (1988). Am. J. Med. 84: 5–14.
Carson, J. L., Strom, B. L., Soper, K. A., West, S. L. and Morse, M. L. (1987). Arch. Int. Med. 147: 85–88.
Caruso, I. and Bianchi Porro, G. (1980). Br. Med. J. 280: 75–78.
Coles, L. S., Fries, J. F., Kraines, R. G. and Roth, S. H. (1983). Am. J. Med. 74: 820–828.
Connor, A. M. and Laposata, M. (1988). Am. J. Clin. Pathol. 89: 216–221.
Doherty, M., Hunt, R. H., Langman, M. J. S., Pounder, R. E., Russell, R. I., Sturrock, R. D. and Thould, A. K. (1987). Ann. Rheum. Dis. 46: 640–643.
Edelson, J. T., Tosteson, A. N. A. and Sax, P. (1990). JAMA 264: 41–47.
Ehsanullah, R. S. B., Page, M. D., Tildesley, G. and Wood, J. R. (1988). Br. Med. J. 297: 1017–1021.
Faulkner, G., Prichard, P., Somerville, K. and Langman, M. J. S. (1988). Br. Med. J. 297: 1311–1313.
Fries, J. F., Miller, S. R., Spitz, P. W., Williams, C. A., Hubert, H. B. and Bloch, D. A. (1989). Gastroenterology 96: 647–655.
Graham, D. Y. and Smith, J. L. (1986). Ann. Intern. Med. 104: 390–398.
Graham, D. Y., Smith, J. L. and Dobbs, S. M. (1988). Dig. Dis. Sci. 28: 1–6.
Graham, D. Y. (1989). Gastroenterology 96: 675–681.
Griffin, M. R., Ray, W. A. and Schaffner, W. (1988). Ann. Intern. Med. 109: 359–363.
Ivey, K. J. (1986). Drugs 32: (suppl. 4). 71–89.
Kurata, J. H. and Abbey, D. E. (1990). J. Clin. Gastroenterol. 12: 260–266.
Langman, M. J. S. (1988). Am. J. Med. 84: 15–19.
Lanas, A., Sekar, M. C., Hirschowitz, B. I. (1991) Gastroenterology 100: A106.
Lussier, A. and LeBel, E. (1987). Am. J. Med. (suppl 4B) 83: 15–18.
McCarthy, D. M. (1989). Gastroenterology 96: 662–674.
Pierson, R. N., Holt, P. R., Watson, R. M. and Keating, R. P. (1961). Am. J. Med. 31: 259–265.
Perrault, J., Fleming, C. R. and Dozois, R. R. (1988). Mayo Clin. Proc. 63: 337–342.
Piper, G. W., Gallatly, R. and McIntosh, J. (1982). Drugs and Peptic Ulcer, vol. 2 (C. J. Pfeiffer, ed.), CRC Press, Boca Raton, FL.
Roth, S. H. (1988). J. Rheumatol. 15: 912–919.
Semble, E. L. and Wu, W. C. (1987). Semin. Arthritis Rheum. 16: 271–286.
Silen, W. (1988). Am. J. Physiol. 255: G395–G402.
Skander, M. P. and Ryan, F. P. (1988). Br. Med. J. 297: 833–834.
Walan, A., Bader, J.-P., Classen, M., Lamers, C. B. H. W., Piper, D. W., Rutgersson, K. and Eriksson, S. (1989). N. Engl. J. Med. 320: 69–74.

Progress in Inflammation
Research and Therapy

Pharmacokinetics, Safety, and Ability to Diminish Leukotriene Synthesis by Zileuton, an Inhibitor of 5-Lipoxygenase

P. Rubin, L. Dubé, R. Braeckman, L. Swanson, R. Hansen, D. Albert, and G. Carter

Abbott Laboratories, One Abbott Park Road, Abbott Park, IL 60064–3500, USA

Summary

Zileuton is a potent and specific inhibitor of 5-lipoxygenase, the first dedicated enzyme in the metabolism of arachidonic acid to the leukotrienes. The leukotrienes have been implicated in numerous pathological conditions. Zileuton was given to normal human volunteers in single doses of 200 mg to 800 mg. Results of these studies indicated that zileuton was well absorbed orally with an elimination half-life of approximately 2.5 hours. Leukotriene B_4 production by ex vivo calcium ionophone stimulated whole blood was inhibited by up to 80% of baseline and correlated with plasma concentrations. Zileuton did not significantly inhibit cyclooxygenase as demonstrated by thromboxane B_2 levels. There were no safety concerns that would preclude development.

Zileuton (N-(1-benzo [b] thien-2-yl)ethyl)-N-hydroxyurea)(A-64077) is a selective 5-lipoxygenase inhibitor with unique anti-inflammatory properties. Because the products of the lipoxygenase pathway, the leukotrienes, have been implicted in the pathophysiology of human disease (Lewis et al., 1990), zileuton may have therapeutic potential in a number of illnesses. The products of the lipoxygenase pathway have been studied in asthma (Arm et al., 1988; Kohi et al., 1990; Takahashi et al., 1988; Arm et al., 1989; Wardlaw et al., 1989) and other pulmonary diseases (Wardlaw et al., 1989; Richards et al., 1989; Stephenson et al., 1988; Davis et al., 1990; Davis et al., 1989), ulcerative colitis and Crohn's disease

(Goetzl et al., 1988; Vilaseca et al., 1990; Schumert et al., 1988; Laursen et al., 1990), rheumatoid arthritis (Sperling et al., 1990), atopic dermatitis (Fogh et al., 1989) and other allergic conditions (Freedland et al., 1989), and ischemic heart disease (Mehta et al., 1989). The present study was designed to achieve the following objectives: (a) to characterize the pharmacokinetics of zileuton in man after a range of single oral doses; (b) to determine whether a relationship exists between the plasma levels of zileuton and its inhibitory activity on leukotriene and thromboxane production; and (c) to evaluate its safety profile.

Methods

Study Design: In this Phase I parallel trial, a total of 36 healthy adult male volunteers were randomized in a double-blind fashion to receive either zileuton or placebo. Subjects received zileuton (200 mg, 400 mg, 600 mg, or 800 mg) or placebo as a single oral dose. Subjects receiving active drug received one or more 200 mg capsules. All subjects fasted for eight hours prior to drug administration and did not eat for an additional four hours post-dose. Heparinized blood was collected for assay prior to and 0.25, 0.5, 0.75, 1, 1.5, 2, 3, 4, 6, 8, 10, 12, 16, 20, 24, 28, 36, 48, and 60 hours after dosing (Tables II and IV, and Figure 1 reflect data from the first 12 hours only).

Blood samples collected for zileuton plasma concentrations were centrifuged and the resultant plasma frozen at $-10°C$ or colder. Blood samples collected for leukotriene (LTB_4) determinations were immediately incubated at 37°C with calcium ionophore (A-23187), a known inducer of leukotriene production in human blood (see assay section below) and then frozen at $-70°C$. Blood samples collected for thromboxane synthesis determination were permitted to coagulate for one hour at 37°C to induce TXA_2 biosynthesis. After centrifuging, serum was collected from these samples and stored frozen until assayed for thromboxane B_2, the stable mebolite of TXA_2.

Chemical Assays: Plasma concentrations of zileuton were determined by high-pressure liquid chromatography using a Spectra-Physics SP8800 Chromatograph equipped with a UV detector set at

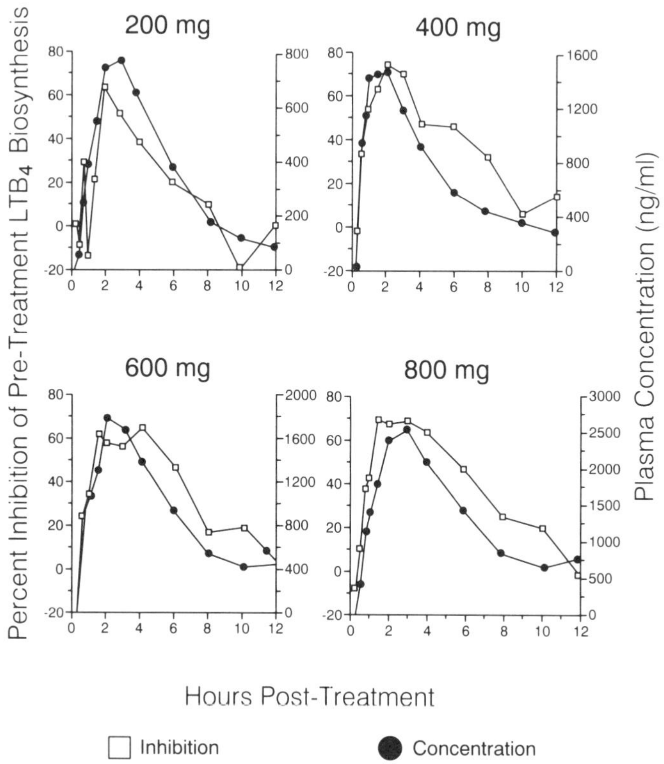

Figure 1. Comparison of LTB_4 inhibition and plasma concentration following oral administration of Abbott-64077.

260nm. Plasma samples were extracted using solid phase C8 columns with diethyl ether as the eluent. The samples were chromatographed on a Supelcosil LC-18 column using a mobile phase consisting of 70% water: 15% acetonitrile: 5% methanol: 10% tetrahydrofuran, containing 40 mM NaH_2PO_4, 7.5 mM H_3PO_4 and 5.0 mM N-aceto-hydroxamic acid.

To evaluate the inhibitory effect of zileuton on 5-lipoxygenase, heparinized blood was incubated for 30 minutes at 37°C with $47 < m < M$ calcium ionophore (A-23187) to trigger LTB_4 biosynthesis. After incubation, the samples were rapidly cooled in an ice bath and then centrifuged at −10°C for 10 minutes. The plasma layers were then removed and stored frozen until assayed. After thawing, plasma samples were mixed with two volumes of methanol and kept at 3°C for 30 minutes prior to centrifugation for an additional 30 minute period. The supernatants were analyzed for LTB_4 with a commercially available radioimmunoassay (RIA) (Amersham, Arlington Heights, Illinois). The linear range of the assay was 10–200 pg per tube.

To evaluate the inhibitory effect of zileuton on cyclooxygenase, thromboxane B_2 (TXB_2) recovered in serum from coagulated blood samples was analyzed in serum samples diluted 1000-fold with RIA buffer using a commercially available RIA kit (Biotex Laboratories, Friendswood, Texas). The linear range of the assay was 1 to 100 pg per tube.

Pharmacokinetic Analysis

The means of the individual observed peak plasma times (T_{max}) and peak concentrations (C_{max}) of zileuton were computed. Individual and mean areas under the concentration-time curves (AUCs) from 0 to 36 hours were calculated using the linear trapezoidal method. The apparent plasma clearance (CI/F, where F represents the bioavailability of the drug) of zileuton was calculated as dose/AUC.

An open one-compartment model was used to determine the pharmacokinetic variables of zileuton. Each parameter value was estimated using a non linear least-squares fitting with NONLIN computer program (Metzler et al., 1974). Means and standard deviations were calculated for each pharmacokinetic parameter.

Statistical Methods: All p-values were based on two-tail tests. P-values less than or equal to 0.05 were considered statistically significant. One-way analysis of variance (one-way ANOVA) was used to compare baseline mean age, height, and weight, as well as all laboratory values.

Mean LTB_4 levels were calculated, as were standard deviations. Changes in LTB_4 levels from time 0 to particular time points were tested within each treatment group by fitting an ANOVA model. Similarly, differences between treatment groups at a given time point were tested using one-way ANOVA for the change from baseline (i.e., time 0) measurements.

LTB_4 values after time 0 were also summarized as percent inhibition relative to LTB_4 formation at time 0 as well as the percent of the time 0 value. Using this methodology, maximum percent inhibition was calculated for each patient. Differences between treatment groups were compared using one-way ANOVA.

Results

There were no significant differences in any demographic parameter except that patients receiving placebo in the 800 mg dose group were significantly older (33.3 ± 2.6 years) than those receiving active medication in the same dose group (25.5 ± 1.8 years [$p < 0.05$]). The overall age ranges for those receiving active drug and those receiving placebo were 18 to 40 years and 19 to 38 years, respectively (Table I).

Mean plasma concentration-time profiles for zileuton after each of the four doses given to the subjects in this study are listed in Table II and shown in Figure 2. Table III lists the pharmacokinetic values calculated for raw data or estimated by the non-linear curve fitting according to the model.

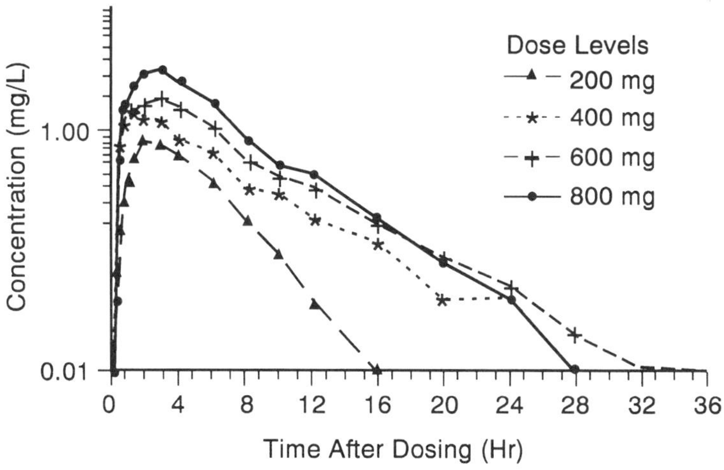

Figure 2. Mean plasma concentrations of Abbott-64077 in man after single oral administration.

Table I. Baseline demographic data

Group	Active Drug (A) or Placebo (P)	Age (yrs)			Height (in)			Weight (lb)		
		Mean	SE	Range	Mean	SE	Range	Mean	SE	Range
I	A (n = 5)	32.2	2.1	29–40	70.4	1.2	67–73	171.6	9.4	146–204
	P (n = 3)	33.0	2.7	28–38	68.8	1.5	67–72	182.6	12.2	166–203
II	A (n = 6)	32.2	3.1	22–40	70.7	1.5	66–75	162.5	8.3	140–184
	P (n = 3)	24.7	4.3	19–30	69.8	2.1	68–73	170.3	11.7	153–195
III	A (n = 6)	28.5	2.3	18–37	69.5	1.8	64–74	163.0	11.0	137–200
	P (n = 3)	25.3	3.2	24–27	69.0	2.5	64–76	155.7	15.5	132–193
IV	A (n = 6)	25.5	1.8	19–32	70.4	1.4	67–75	168.7	8.7	142–201
	P (n = 3)	33.3*	2.6	29–37	70.7	2.0	66–74	148.8	12.4	142–156

Group I: 200 mg or placebo. Group II: 400 mg or placebo. Group III: 600 mg or placebo. Group IV: 800 mg or placebo.
*$p < 0.05$ between active drug and placebo

Table II. Plasma concentrations of zileuton after administration of single oral doses

Dose	*Concentration (mg/l)* *Hours after oral administration*												
	0	0.25	0.5	0.75	1.0	1.5	2.0	3.0	4.0	6.0	8.0	10.0	12.0
200 mg	0.00	0.00	0.07	0.26	0.38	0.55	0.83	0.70	0.64	0.40	0.19	0.10	0.04
400 mg	0.00	0.08	0.80	1.17	1.33	1.43	1.34	1.24	0.88	0.67	0.34	0.29	0.19
600 mg	0.00	0.08	0.58	1.04	1.24	1.50	1.64	1.90	1.65	1.10	0.58	0.42	0.34
800 mg	0.00	0.01	0.57	1.51	1.65	2.23	2.95	3.20	2.63	1.75	0.90	0.52	0.43

Table III. Pharmacokinetic parameters of zileuton following single doses in man (all values as mean ± S.D.)

	Dose of Zileuton			
	200 *mg*	400 *mg*	600 *mg*	800 *mg*
T_{max}	2.5 ± 1.0	1.8 ± 1.1	2.5 ± 0.8	2.3 ± 0.9
C_{max}	0.91 ± 0.26	1.75 ± 0.44	2.07 ± 0.92	3.42 ± 0.77
Ka	1.32 ± 0.91	3.68 ± 2.94	1.07 ± 1.01	1.41 ± 1.68
Ke	0.33 ± 0.05	0.29 ± 0.08	0.31 ± 0.15	0.30 ± 0.08
$T_{1/2}$	2.10 ± 0.35	2.38 ± 0.71	2.22 ± 1.21	2.29 ± 0.61
V/F	145 ± 38	186 ± 68	189 ± 99	148 ± 59
AUC	4.43 ± 0.76	9.37 ± 2.00	13.78 ± 2.49	21.61 ± 5.38
Cl/F	770 ± 129	741 ± 164	748 ± 150	689 ± 199

Abbreviations: see text units: T_{max}, $T_{1/2}$, (hr); C_{max} (mg/L); AUC (mg·hr/L); Cl/F (mL/min); Ka, Ke (hr^{-1}); V/F (L).
Note: the pharmacokinetic parameters were determined by nonlinear curve-fitting, as determined from the model. Half-lives are presented as harmonic means and pseudo standard deviations.

Plasma concentrations of zileuton peaked at 1 to 3 hours after dosing. Mean peak plasma concentrations (C_{max}) following single 200 mg, 400 mg, 600 mg, and 800 mg doses were 0.91, 1.75. 2.07. and 3.42 mg/L, respectively. The absorption of zileuton showed large interpatient variability, with K_a values ranging from 1.1 to 3.7 hr^{-1}.

Following peak plasma concentrations, zileuton plasma levels decreased with a mean elimination half-life of 2.3 hours. The half-life was independent of dose. The overall mean apparent plasma clearance was 737 mL/min, which was also dose-independent. Similarly, the mean apparent volume of distribution (V/F) – 167 liters – was also dose-independent. The mean AUC increased linearly from 4.43 mg·hr/L with the 200 mg dose to 20.61 mg·hr/L with the 800 mg dose.

Leukotriene and Thromboxane Synthesis

Blood collected from subjects given zileuton had a significantly reduced capacity to synthesize LTB_4 in response to A-23187 as compared with placebo or baseline. The reduction was most pronounced 1.5 to 4 hours post-dose (Table IV). The mean maximum individual percent reduction of LTB_4 biosynthesis was 72%, 82%, 76%, and 82% after 200 mg, 400 mg, 600 mg, and 800 mg doses, respectively. Thus, the mean effect appeared to have reached a plateau at the 400 mg dosage. The duration of statistically significant inhibition was extended from 2 hours with the 200 mg dose to a range of 5.0 to 7.5 hours with the higher doses. The onset of statistically significant inhibition, as compared with baseline activity, was 2.0 hours with the 200 mg dose and 0.5 to 1.0 hour with higher doses.

The relationship between the extent of inhibition of LTB_4 and plasma concentration of zileuton is shown in Figure 1. The LTB_4 inhibition profile correlates significantly with the plasma profile of zileuton after each dose.

There was no consistent effect of zileuton on cyclooxygenase inhibition, as assessed by TXB_2 concentrations. No significant differences from baseline values were observed, with the singular exception of the 12-hour sample following the 200 mg dose (TXB_2 level significantly higher than placebo [$p < 0.05$]).

Safety

The study of zileuton was assessed by analysis of tabulated adverse events and changes from pre-study values in vital signs, body weight, electrocardiograms, and laboratory test results. As compared with placebo, statistically significant elevations were rarely seen and were not of clinical significance. For example , the Day 2 determination of SGPT (ALT) following the 400 mg dose demonstrated a minor 5.1 IU/L elevation following zileuton as compared to a 2.8 IU/L reduction after placebo ($p < 0.05$). Thus, there were no meaningful alterations in chemistry, coagulation, or hematologic laboratory parameters, hormone and gonadotropin levels, creatinine clearance determinations, semen sample evaluations, electrocardiography, electroencephalography, or vital signs.

Three subjects – 1 given a 200 mg, 1 given a 400 mg, and 1 given placebo – had elevations in SGPT to values greater than the upper limit of normal. One of the three (the one given the 200 mg) had an

Table IV. Inhibition of leukotriene B5 (LTB_4) biosynthesis in whole blood after administration of single doses of zileuton or placebo (figures expressed as mean percent of pre-dose levels)

	Hours after oral administration											
Dose	0.25	0.5	0.75	1.0	1.5	2.0	3.0	4.0	6.0	8.0	0.0	12.0
Placebo	112	100	117	120	105	105	129[a]	137[a]	134[a]	136[a]	140[a]	124
200 mg	101	107	71[b]	114	79[b]	37[c]	49[c]	62[c]	81[b]	91	123	101
400 mg	102	67[c]	47[c]	47[c]	38[c]	27[c]	31[c]	54[c]	55[c]	68[c]	94[b]	87[b]
600 mg	121	75	76[b]	65[c]	37[c]	41[c]	43[c]	34[c]	53[c]	83[b]	81[b]	97[b]
800 mg	108	89	61[c]	57[c]	30[c]	31[c]	30[c]	35[c]	53[c]	75[c]	91[b]	101

[a] Values differ significantly ($p < 0.05$) from baseline (pre-dose) levels.
[b] Values differ significantly ($p < 0.05$) from placebo at the corresponding time.
[c] Values differ significantly ($p < 0.05$) from baseline levels and from placebo at the corresponding time.

elevated SGOT at baseline (77 IU/L; normal range: 6 to 59) but no further significant increase occurred during therapy. A patient receiving a 400 mg dose experienced a pre-dose increase in SGPT from 30 to 53 IU/L between Day 11 and Day 1; SGPT continued to increase to 72, 84, 105, and 127 IU/L, on Days 2, 3, 4, and 7, respectively. Unfortunately, this subject was lost to follow-up. A placebo recipient experienced elevated SGPT levels of 76 and 85 IU/L on Day 3 and Day 4, respectively; levels fell to within the normal range by Day 14. Neither one of these last two subjects had any other laboratory abnormality or clinical signs or symptoms associated with SGPT elevations. However, both subjects had significant IgM titers to cytomegalovirus four days after dosing, suggesting acute CMV infection as opposed to true drug effect.

Mild nausea, "upset stomach", "stomachache", mild lower abdominal pain, and "queasy stomach" were reported by a total of 5 subjects, 4 of whom received active drug. All resolved without treatment. Headache and fatigue were reported in subjects given active drug and placebo.

Discussion

The release of arachidonic acid from cell membrane phospholipids in response to the activity of phospholipase A_2 results in the production of a family of compounds known as eicosanoids (Lewis et al., 1990). Subsequent degradation of arachidonic acid via the cyclooxygenase pathway results in the production of prostaglandins and thromboxanes, whereas degradation via the 5-lipoxygenase pathway results in a large family of compounds known as leukotrienes (Lewis et al., 1990).

There is a wide and growing body of literature on the role of leukotrienes in human disease. Neutrophils isolated from patients with exercise-induced asthma are hyperresponsive in their ability to produce leukotriene B_4(LTB_4) during an acute episode (Arm et al., 1988). LTC_4 (Kohi et al., 1990) and LTB_4 (Takahashi et al., 1988) generation has been demonstrated to be greater in asthmatics, symptomatic asthmatics, and patients with allergic rhinitis than in normal controls (Wardlaw et al., 1989). Patients with aspirin-induced asthma show a marked airway responsiveness to LTE_4 (Arm et al, 1989). The administration of a selective LTB_4 antagonist (U-75302) has been shown to reduce eosinophil adherence to bronchiolar capillaries in an animal model of bronchopulmonary eosinophilia (Stephenson et al., 1988). Leukotriene involvement has also been demonstrated in patients with or at risk for adult respitatory distress syndrome and other forms of pulmonary failure (Davis et al., 1990; Davis et al., 1989; Goetzl et al., 1988).

Elevated levels of leukotrienes as well as other eicosanoids can be found in the lesional fluids of patients with inflammatory bowel disease (Vilaseca et al., 1990; Schumert et al., 1988). Concentrations of LTB_4 rise quickly in experimental colitis (Laursen et al., 1990), and importantly, agents which reduce LTB_4 concentrations also reduce inflammation (Schumert et al., 1988; Sperling et al., 1990). Recently, zileuton (A-64077) given as a single 800 mg dose to 10 patients with active ulcerative colitis caused a marked reduction in LTB_4 concentrations in rectal dialysis fluid that was sustained for 8 hours, leading to speculation that this drug may play a major anti-inflammatory role in ulcerative colitis (Laursen et al., 1990).

Zileuton is a selective 5-lipoxygenase inhibitor with no significant effect on the cyclooxygenase pathway. The present study was designed to elucidate the pharmacokinetics, pharmacodynamics, and safety profile of this interesting new drug. Zileuton was absorbed rapidly after oral administration of 200 mg to 800 mg single doses. The elimination half-life of zileuton is short (2.3 hours) due to a large apparent clearance (737 mL/min) and a moderate apparent volume of distribution (167 L). The high clearance suggests very rapid intrinsic metabolism and/or first-pass elimination of the drug. The study demonstrated that the elimination half-life, apparent clearance, and apparent volume of distribution of zileuton are dose-independent, indicative of linear pharmacokinetics.

Zileuton administration was associated with a significantly diminished degree of biosynthesis of LTB_4 in response to A-23187. The maximal effect occurred at 1.5 to 4 hours post-dose. The mean effect and the duration of the effect appeared to have reached a plateau at the 400 mg dosage. There was a significant association between the degree of LTB_4 inhibition and zileuton plasma concentrations. There was no consistent effect of zileuton on cyclooxygenase inhibition, as assessed by TXB_2 concentrations. Thus, the study demonstrated the selective inhibition of zileuton on the 5-lipoxygenase side of arachidonic acid metabolism.

There were no meaningful alterations in chemistry, coagulation, or hematologic laboratory parameters, hormone and gonadotropin levels, creatinine clearance determinations, semen sample evaluations, electrocardiography, electroencephalography, or vital signs. Thus, based on this preliminary trial, zileuton appears to be a safe drug which selectively and effectively inhibits 5-lipoxygenase, and holds potential value for the treatment of several human diseases.

References

Arm, J. P., O'Hickey, S. P., Spur, B. W. et al. (1989). Airway responsiveness to histamine and leukotriene E_4 in subjects with aspirin-induced asthma. Am. Rev. Resp. Dis. 140: 148–153.

Arm, J. P., Horton, C. E., House, T. J. H. et al. (1988). Enhanced generation of leukotriene B_4 by neutrophils stimulated by unopsonized zymosan and by calcium ionophore after exercise-induced asthma. Am. Rev. Resp. Dis. 138: 47–53.

Davis, J. M., Meyer, J. D., Barie, P. S. et al. (1990). Elevated production of neutrophil leukotriene B_4 precedes pulmonary failure in critically ill surgical patients. Surg. Gynecol. Obstet. 170: 495–500.

Davis, J. M., Yurt, R. W., Barie, P. S. et al. (1989). Leukotriene B_4 generation in patients with established pulmonary failure. Arch. Surg. 124: 1451–1455

Fogh, K., Herlin, T., Kragballe, K. (1989). Eicosanoids in skin of patients with atopic dermatitis: prostaglandin E_2 and leukotriene B_4 are present in biologically active concentrations. J. Allergy. Clin. Immunol. 83: 450–455.

Freeland, H. S., Pipkorn, U., Schleimer, R. P. et al. (1989). Leukotriene B_4 as a mediator of early and late reactions to antigen in humans: the effect of systemic glucocorticoid treatment in vivo. J. Allergy. Clin. Immunol. 83: 634–642,

Goetzl, E. J., Burrall, B. A., Baud, L. et al. (1988). Generation and recognition of leukotriene mediators of hypersensitivity and inflammation. Dig. Dis. Sci. 33: (suppl) 36S–40S.

Kohi, F., Miyagawa, H., Agrawal, D. K. et al. (1990). Generation of leukotriene B_4 and C_4 from granulocytes of normal controls, allergic rhinitis, and asthmatic subjects. Ann. Allergy. 65: 228–232.

Lewis, R. A., Austen, K. F., Soberman, R. J. (1990). Leukotrienes and other products of the 5-lipoxygenase pathway. Biochemistry and relation to pathobiology in human disease. N. Engl. J. Med. 323: 645–655.

Laursen, L. S., Naesdal, J., Bukhave, K. et al. (1990). Selective 5-lipoxygenase inhibition in ulcerative colitis. Lancet. 333: 683–685.

Mehta, J., Dinerman, J., Mehta, P. et al. (1989). Neutrophil function in ischemic heart disease. Circulation. 79: 549–556.

Metzler, C. M., Elfring, G. L., McEwen, A. J. (1974). A package of computer programs for pharmacokinetic modeling. Biometrics. 30: 562–563.

Richards, I. M., Griffin, R. L., Oostveen, J. A. et al. (1989). Effect of the selective leukotriene B_4 antagonist U-75302 on antigen-induced bronchopulmonary eosinophilia in sensitized guinea pigs. Am. Rev. Resp. Dis. 140: 1712–1718.

Schumert, R., Towner, J., Zipser, R. D. (1988). Role of eicosanoids in human and experimental colitis. Dig. Dis. Sci., 33: (suppl) 58S–64S.

Sperling, R. I., Coblyn, J. S., Larkin, J. K. et al. (1990). Inhibition of leukotriene B_4 synthesis in neutrophils from patients with rheumatoid arthritis by a single oral dose of methotrexate. Arth. Rheumat. 33: 1149–1155.

Stephenson, A. H., Lonigro, A. J., Hyers, T. M. et al. (1988). Increased concentrations of leukotrienes in bronchoalveolar lavage fluid of patients with ARDS or at risk for ARDS. Am. Rev. Resp. Dis. 138: 714–719.

Takahashi, K., Shimizu, I., Kimura, I. et al. (1988). Production of leukotrienes and superoxide from neutrophil-rich fraction of bronchial asthmatics. Jpn. J. Allergol. 37: 322–330.

Vilaseca, J., Salas, A., Guarner, F. et al. (1990). Participation of thromboxane and other eicosanoid synthesis in the course of experimental inflammatory colitis. Gastroenterology. 98: 269–277.

Wardlaw, A. J., Hay, H., Cromwell, O. et al. (1989). Leukotrienes, LTC_4 and LTB_4 in bronchoalveolar lavage in bronchial asthma and other respiratory diseases. J. Allergy. Clin. Immunol. 84: 19–26.

AAS 35
Progress in Inflammation
Research and Therapy

Combined DMARDS in Rheumatoid Arthritis: Past, Present and Future

D. E. Yocum,

Department of Internal Medicine, Arizona Arthritis Center, University of Arizona, Tucson, AZ 84724, USA

Summary

The potential for combined therapy in rheumatoid arthritis is rapidly increasing considering the recent development of various new treatment modalities. However, an aggressive effort must be made to stage patients according to various clinical and immunological parameters. Only then can appropriate combined therapy be used effectively in this disease process. The development of such combined therapy could expand into other diseases such as scleroderma, systemic lupus erythematosus and multiple sclerosis.

Rheumatoid arthritis is a disease of unknown etiology and with no known cure characterized by a chronic proliferative and erosive synovitis that waxes and wanes over the lifetime of the effected individual. It typically presents in the third and fourth decade in life and is associated with significant morbidity and mortality resulting in hospitalizations and significant medical costs. Recent data demonstrates that progressive rheumatoid arthritis has a worse prognosis than Hodgkins lymphoma.

In spite of the significant costs to the patients and society, little progress has been made in developing new treatments for this disease. To date, single agent therapy has had limited effect, typically with less than one-third of patients remaining on an individual treatment after one year (Amor et al., 1981). While greater numbers of patients are remaining on methotrexate therapy past one year, very few patients achieve remission (Williams et al., 1985). There has been a growing commitment over the last five years to develop appropriate and effective combination therapy. Lessons from oncology have taught physicians that combined drug therapy results not only in more effective treatment with greater remissions but also less toxicity to individual drugs.

There have been very limited attempts at combination therapy in the past. Most of these have dealt with using combinations of the standard disease modifying drugs (Tiliakos, 1986; Bunch et al., 1984; Csuka et al., 1986). Not only have many of these studies been very poorly designed, but the numbers of patients and the data collected from these studies are hard to evaluate, ultimately reported only in abstract form. There can be no clear cut decisions made from these studies and considering that the mechanism of action of this group of drugs is so poorly delineated, future work with combining these agents will probably provide very little information. However, these studies demonstrate how important it is to develop well organized studies with suitable numbers of patients entered.

Recently more aggressive combinations of drugs have been tried. The two most notable studies involve the use of combination cytotoxic therapy. The first done was an open study in which over 30 patients with severe refractory rheumatoid arthritis were treated with a combination of cyclophosphamide, azathioprine and hydroxychloroquine (Csuka et al., 1986). However, while over three-quarters of these patients either achieved remission or had a very positive response, they had an exceedingly high rate of neoplasia and death secondary to infection. This study suggested that appropriate combination therapy could be more effective than our standard single agent therapy, but combining two or more cytotoxic agents may result in undue morbidity and mortality. More recently from the Cleveland Clinic, a study of the use of combined methotrexate and azathioprine has been done (Biro et al., 1987). The initial pilot study suggested that this combination may be more effective than either drug individually. There is presently an ongoing multicenter study looking at this combination.

The future of combination therapy and rheumatoid arthritis depends upon appropriate use of the present understanding of the pathophysiology of this disease. Better use of available research information on this disease will help guide future combined therapy. It is clear that we can identify the patients who present with rheumatoid arthritis who will have a poor prognosis. Too frequently patients with different clinical presentations, different disease duration and different histology are grouped together into multicenter studies. The wide variability of response in these studies demonstrates the heterogeneity of the patients entered into the studies. In addition to the clinical data, recent information demonstrates that at least two histologic groups of rheumatoid arthritis patients exists (Malone et al., 1984). The first group which is characterized by lymphocyte infiltrated tissue is associated with peripheral blood hypoproliferation to soluble recall antigens (Haraoui et al., 1984). The other group, characterized by more fibrin and scar formation have peripheral blood lymphocytes which respond normally to recall antigens. Not only are the hypo-proliferative group more likely to have heavy T cell infiltrates into their tissue, but, they also have a lower peripheral blood helper/suppressor ratio, spontaneously produce greater amounts of rheumatoid factor, have elevated levels of natural killer cells and lack natural killer cell regulation of B cell proliferation. In addition, recent data by Yocum, et al., (Arthritis Rheum, in press) demonstrates as did previous work by others that anergic patients are more likely to respond to immunomodulation with such agents as cyclosporin or with leukapheresis (Wahl et al., 1983).

The development of monoclonal antibodies, especially the humanized and chimeric type as well as new advances in molecular biology have provided us with a wide array of new, potentially very useful tools in treating rheumatoid arthritis in a combined fashion (Herzog et al., 1989). Such treatment modalities as anti-CD5, anti-CD4, anti-MHC Class II, anti-IL2 receptor, anti-T cell receptor, pseudomonas exotoxin conjugates and the production of various biologics in massive quantities are a few of the recent treatments developed. In addition to this, the number of immunomodulatory drugs available has expanded greatly. Agents such as rapamyacin and FK506 represent new additions to cyclosporin.

Therefore, by using the available information that we have concerning clinical and basic data on those patients who are more likely to progress and the subgroups of these patients should help us to direct combined therapy. While each of these modalities will have to be tested on its own merits, each alone should not be heavily criticized for any lack of efficacy but only excessive amounts of toxicity. The real key to these treatments lies in the ability to combine them with two or more medications. Preliminary data has demonstrated positive effects in a study using a combination of cyclosporin and methotrexate in rheumatoid arthritis. While it appears effective here, other authors feel that this combination may be ineffective in other diseases such as psoriatic arthritis. Therefore, individual diseases will have to be evaluated and the positive or negative results cannot be assumed in another disease. Finally, early disease (less than one year in duration) needs to be separated from early progressive disease (established erosions without deformity) and end stage disease (significant erosions and deformities).

Using such data, an appropriate program in early rheumatoid arthritis might be to use pulses of humanized monoclonal anti-CD4 alternating with a pseudomonas exotoxin conjugate with IL-2 in combination with an IL-1 inhibitor and/or cyclosporin. The goal here would be to shut down the early cascade of inflammatory events that occur from the macrophage and the T cell. Not all of these agents would be given at once and would be used in sequence to more effectively suppress the abnormal immune response. In contrast, in later established disease, a possible combination of treatments may be to use humanized monoclonal anti-MHC Class 2 or anti-TNF antibodies in addition to a pseudomonas exotoxin conjugate with a growth factor with receptors limited to synovial fibroblasts and/or another treatment with an agent such as methotrexate to slow the proliferative process. Cyclosporin could be added to those patients who exhibit hypoproliferative responses to recall antigens.

Conclusion

The potential for combined therapy in rheumatoid arthritis is vast considering the recent development of various new treatment modalities. However, a very aggressive effort must be made to appropriately categorize or stage patients according to various clinical and immunological parameters. Only then can appropriate combined therapy potentially be used effectively in this disease process. The development of such combined therapy would then open into a host of diseases such as scleroderma, systemic lupus erythematosus and multiple sclerosis.

References

Amor, B., Herson, D., Cherot, A. and Delbarre, F. (1981). Follow-up study of patients with rheumatoid arthritis over a period of more than 10 years (1966–1978): analysis of disease progression and treatment in 100 cases, Ann. Med. Interne. 132: 168–173.

Biro, J. A., Segal, A. M., MacKenzie, A. H., Mazanec, D. J. and Wilke, W. S. (1987). The combination of methotrexate and azathioprine for resistant rheumatoid arthritis, Arthritis Rheum. 30: S18.

Bunch, T. W., O'Duffy, J. D., Tompkins, R. B. and O'Fallon, W. M. (1984). Controlled trial of hydroxychloroquine and D-penicillamine singly and in combination in the treatment of rheumatoid arthritis, Arthritis Rheum. 27: 267.

Csuka, M., Carreara, G. F. and McCarty, D. J. (1986). Treatment of intractable rheumatoid arthritis with combined cyclophosphamide, azathioprine and hydroxychloroquine: A follow-up study. JAMA. 255: 2315–2319.

Haraoui, B., Wilder, R. L., Malone, D. G., Allen, J. B., Katona, I. M. and Wahl, S. M. (1984). Immune function in severe, active rheumatoid arthritis: A relationship between peripheral blood mononuclear cell proliferation to soluble antigens and mononuclear cell subset profiles. J. Immunol. 133: 697–701.

Herzog, C., Walker, C., Muller, W., Rieger, P., Reiter, C., Reithmuller, G., Wassmer, P., Stockinger, H., Madic, O. and Pichler, W. J. (1989). Anti-$CD4^+$ antibody treatment of patients with rheumatoid arthritis: I. Effect on clinical and circulating T cells, J. Autoimm. 2: 627–642.

Malone, D. Gl., Wahl, S. M., Tsokos, M., Cattell, H., Decker, J. L. and Wilder, R. L. (1984). Immune function in severe active rheumatoid arthritis: A relationship between peripheral blood mononuclear cell proliferation to soluble antigens and synovial tissue immunohistologic characteristics, J. Clin. Invest. 74: 1173–1185.

Tiliakos, N. A. (1986). Low-dose cytotoxic drug combination therapy in intractable rheumatoid arthritis: Two years later, Arthritis Rheum. 29: S79.

Wahl, S. M., Wilder, R. L., Katona, I. M., Wahl, L. M., Allen, J. B., Scher, I. and Decker, J. L. (1983). Leukapheresis in rheumatoid arthritis: Association of clinical improvement with reversal of anergy, Arthritis Rheum. 26: 1076–1084.

Williams, H. J., Willkens, R. F., Samuelson, C. O., Alarcon, G. S., Guttadauria, M., Yarboro, C., Polisson, R. P., Weiner, S. R., Luggen, M. E., Billingsley, L. M., Dahl, S. L., Egger, M. J., Reading, J. C. and Ward, J. R. (1985). Comparison of low-dose oral pulse methotrexate and placebo in the treatment of rheumatoid arthritis. A Controlled Clinical Trial, Arthritis Rheum. 28: 721–730.

Workshop Sessions

AAS 35
Progress in Inflammation
Research and Therapy

Design and Development of Drugs

R. M. McMillan and G. W. Carter***

*Bioscience I, ICI Pharmaceuticals, Mereside, Alderley Park, Macclesfield, Cheshire, SK10 4TG, U.K. and **Abbott Laboratories, Department 462, AP9, Abbott Park, IL 60064, U.S.A.

Therapy in the majority of chronic inflammatory diseases is inadequate with current drugs suffering from either insufficient efficacy, serious toxicity or both. Thus, discovery of new drugs that control inflammatory symptoms or modulate disease activity continues to be an area of intense activity in the pharmaceutical industry. The workshop on "Design and Development of Drugs" at the Fifth International Meeting of the Inflammation Research Association reviewed progress in a number of novel drug areas. The objective of the workshop was to review case histories of potential drugs based on a variety of biological targets. These ranged from modulators of lipid mediators, through inhibitors of proteinases and cytokine release to novel immunomodulators. Most of the drugs were in or about to enter clinical trials at the time of the workshop and, where appropriate, their clinical status is described below.

A. Antagonism of Lipid Mediators

In view of the wide range of biological actions exhibited by leukotrienes considerable activity has centered on development of drugs that inhibit their synthesis or actions. Lipoxygenase inhibitors and antagonists of peptido-leukotrienes are currently undergoing clinical evaluation. Dr. S. W. Djuric (G. D. Searle) discussed SC-41930 which is the first LTB_4 receptor antagonist to reach clinical evaluation. The discovery of SC-41930 [Djuric et al.] repre-

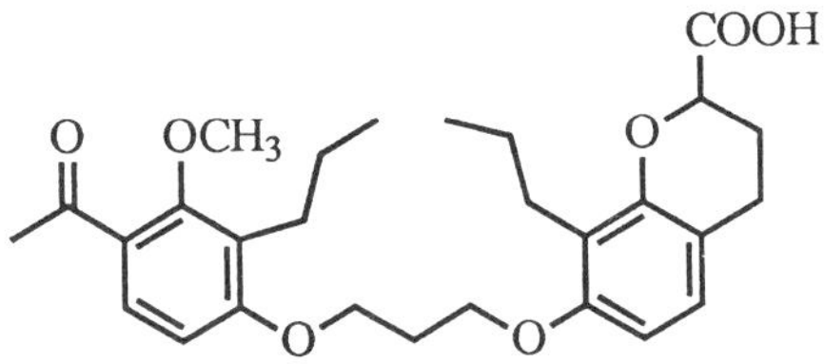

SC-41930

sented an example of a "semi-rational" lead seeking approach. In the absence of a published lead agent, the Searle peptido-leukotriene antagonist database was screened for compounds with LTB_4 antagonist activity. This led to the discovery of SC-41930 which prevented LTB_4 receptor binding to human neutrophils with an IC_{50} of 0.3 μM. Following a novel resolution procedure, the (+) and (−) enantiomers of SC-41930 were found to be equiactive *in vitro* and subsequent studies concentrated on the racemate. SC-41930 was at least 50 times more potent as an antagonist of LTB_4 than of LTD_4 and was 10 times more potent at inhibiting responses to LTB_4 than FMLP. *In vivo*, SC-41930 potently inhibited LTB_4-induced chemotaxis in guinea pig skin ($ED_{50} = 0.6$ mg/kg, p.o.) but, surprisingly, was much less potent in inhibiting chemotaxis induced by 12R-HETE which is believed to mediate its actions via the LTB_4 receptor. Since SC-41930 is being developed for ulcerative colitis and psoriasis, it was encouraging that the compound also demonstrated activity in models of skin inflammation and colitis. SC-41930 is currently in Phase I studies and exhibits a half-life in man of approximately 6 hours.

Continuing the theme of lipid mediators, Dr. W. H. Parsons (Merck) reviewed the development of orally-active antagonists of platelet activating factor (PAF). It is well established that the biological actions of PAF extend well beyond the platelet and therapeutic potential for PAF antagonists has been proposed in a wide range of inflammatory disorders. The Merck program began in 1982 and initially focused on the natural product kadsurenone which displayed potent PAF antagonism. Concurrently, veraguensin, a structurally-related product which was originally isolated from a Mexican tree, was also shown to be a PAF antagonist *in vitro* ($IC_{50} = 1.1$ μM in rabbit platelet membranes).

Medicinal Chemistry at Merck focussed on seeking orally-active analogues of veraguensin. This effort led to the identification of L-652,731 which was approximately 100 times more potent than veraguensin in the rabbit platelet binding assay ($IC_{50} = 9$ nM) but the compound had limited oral activity due to rapid metabolism.

The antagonist potency was improved a further 10 fold with L-659,989 and potent oral activity was observed in female rats. However, oral activity was very poor in the male due to gender-dependent metabolism; the half-life in females was approximately 3 hours but was less than 20 min in males. Efforts to block metabolism led to the development of MK287 [Sahoo, et al.], which retained potent *in vitro* antagonism of PAF (IC_{50} values of 3–6 nM in platelets and PMN) and showed improved *in vivo* activity. There was still a sex difference in oral activity with MK287 in the rat ($ED_{50} = 0.1$ and 2.3 mg/kg in female and male respectively against PAF-induced plasma extravasation). Extravasation was blocked for up to 7 hours with 1 mg/kg MK287 and the compound also blocked LPS-induced hypotension. In pulmonary systems, MK287 blocked PAF-induced bronchoconstriction and inhibited late phase reactions in allergic sheep. MK287 is currently in Phase II trials in asthma.

B. Inhibition of Collagenase

Neutral proteinases, particularly collagenases, are believed to play a key role in the pathogenesis of a variety of clinical conditions including arthritis, periodontal disease, metastases and corneal ulceration. Dr. M. Crimmin (British Biotechnology) described the evolution of a series of collagenase inhibitors which arose from a transatlantic collaboration between British Biotechnology and SmithKline Beecham. Although no X-ray structure is available for collagenases, the mechanism and site of action of this class of enzymes is well defined [Johnson et al.]. Tissue collagenase has a neutral pH optimum, contains zinc in its active site and is highly specific for collagen, cleaving the 3 chains of the triple helix at a single point approximately three quarters of the way along the molecule. The cleavage site is either glycine-leucine or glycine isoleucine depending on the collagen type.

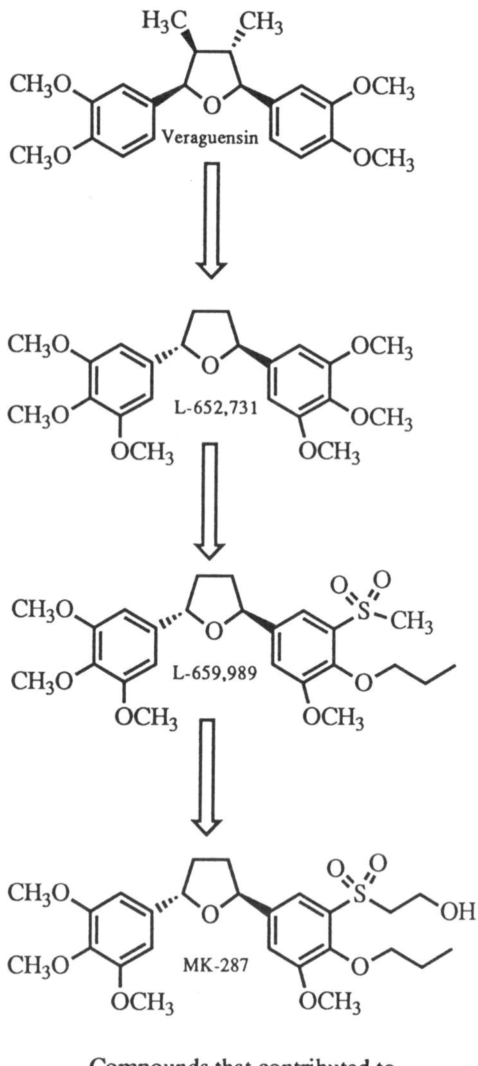

Compounds that contributed to the discovery of MK-287.

Initial drug design involved introduction of zinc chelating functions (e.g. hydroxamic acids, thiols, phosphonic acids) into peptides based on the sequence around the collagen cleavage site. This yielded valuable information on the structural requirements for collagenase inhibition which led to the design of pseudopeptides containing a

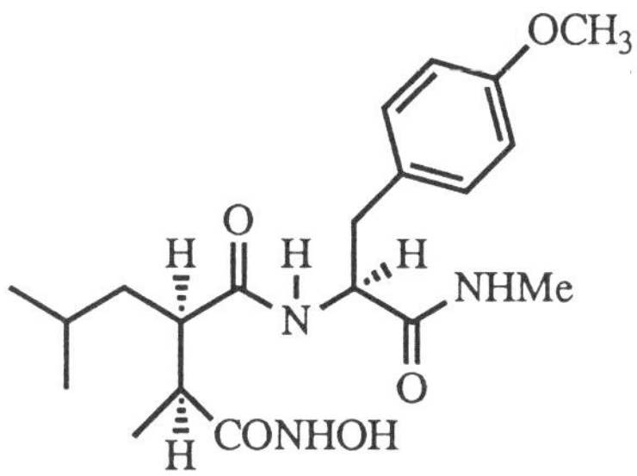

BB16

hydroxamate chelating group. Introduction of a methyl substituent alpha to the hydroxamate yielded optically active compounds. Flexible, stereoselective synthetic routes were developed and this allowed the demonstration that collagenase inhibition was predominantly associated with the R-diastereomer, BB16 ($IC_{50} = 5$ nM), whilst the S-diastereomer, BB15, was much less potent ($IC_{50} > 1$ μM). Similar stereo-selective activity was observed *in vivo*: BB16 (5 mg/kg, i.p.) significantly inhibited paw swelling in adjuvant arthritic rats whereas BB15 was inactive at 20 mg/kg. In addition, histomorphological studies indicated significant bone and cartilage sparing effects of BB16. These data support the anti-arthritic potential of collagenase inhibitors and provide valuable pharmacological probes but, unfortunately, the compounds discussed were not orally active. No inhibitors are yet suitable as clinical candidates but preliminary safety studies indicate no overt toxicity at doses up to 100 mg/kg i.p.

C. Modulation of IL-1 Release

In contrast to the highly specific targets of the earlier talks, Dr. T. Payne (Sandoz) reviewed the biological properties of IX 207-887, an agent which was initially of interest because of its desirable anti-arthritic profile in animal models but subsequently has been shown to inhibit release of IL-1. The initial target of the Sandoz program was discovery of anti-rheumatic agents that did not mediate their actions via inhibition of cyclo-oxygenase. IX 207-887 [Schnyder, et al.] inhibited adjuvant arthritis when dosed therapeutically ($ED_{50} = 12$ mg/kg, p.o.) and had comparable potency against *E.*

coli.-induced fever and LPS-induced acute phase response ($ED_{50} \sim 20$ mg/kg, p.o.). The compound did not inhibit cyclo-oxygenase, 5-lipoxygenase or PLA_2 *in vitro* and did not inhibit cyclo-oxygenase dependent responses *in vivo*: castor oil diarrhea in rat, *ex vivo* platelet aggregation in rabbit and guinea pig, or PGE_2 release from rabbit gastric mucosa. Moreover, IX 207-887 was not ulcerogenic at doses up to 500 mg/kg p.o., and its major metabolite (the 10-keto derivative) was not a cyclo-oxygenase inhibitor. Prolonged dosing of IX 207-887 in adjuvant arthritis led to more pronounced inhibition of paw swelling with over 50% inhibition detected at daily doses down to 2.5 mg/kg at 20–30 days. Doses in the same range where paw swelling was inhibited prevented the development of histological changes and decreased alpha 2 macroglobulin levels. Very high plasma levels of drug were achieved with therapeutic dosing. Thus, peak and trough levels of 660 and 77 μM, respectively, were detected following administration of 30 mg/kg/day in dog and similar values have subsequently been obtained with therapeutically effective doses in man. Studies *in vitro* demonstrated that these levels of IX 207-887 inhibit LPS-induced release of IL-1 from mononuclear cells. The compound was a weaker inhibitor of IL-6 and TNF alpha release but LPS-induced synthesis of PGE_2 was inhibited at the same concentrations as IL-1 release which is of interest in view of the absence of cyclo-oxygenase inhibition. IX 207-887 also inhibited LPS-induced PGE_2 synthesis *in vivo* in an air pouch model. Whilst the precise mechanism is unknown, it appears that the compound selectively inhibits secretion of inflammatory mediators from macrophages. IX 207-887 is currently in Phase II trials in rheumatoid arthritis.

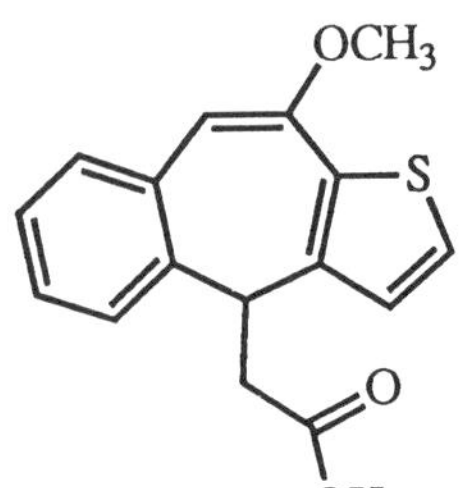

IX 207-887

D. Immunosuppressants

The general belief that rheumatoid arthritis is an auto-immune disease coupled with the recent demonstration that cyclosporin A is efficacious against this crippling disease has stimulated the search for novel immunomodulators with improved safety profiles. The final speakers in the workshop discussed two of the more promising new agents in this area, FK506 and rapamycin.

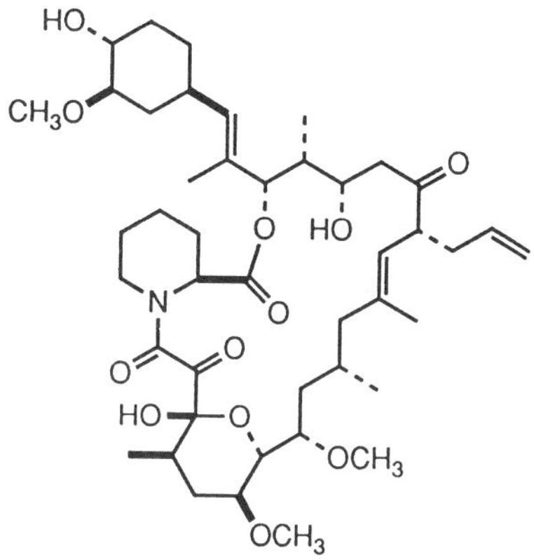

FK-506

Dr. A. Blackham (Fisons) discussed the profile of the macrolide FK506, a fungal metabolite which was first discovered at Fujisawa Pharmaceuticals in Japan [Kino, et al.]. FK506 is approximately 100 times more potent than cyclosporin A in inhibiting mixed lymphocyte reactions *in vitro*. The proposed mode of action of FK506 involves binding to a cytosolic protein termed $FK506_{bp}$, which possesses peptide prolyl isomerase (PPIase) activity as does the cyclosporin A binding protein, cyclophilin [Siekierka]. FK506 is currently in Phase II clinical trials with transplant patients as the initial target. Unless serious toxicity is encountered in these studies, it is likely that clinical development will follow a similar path to cyclosporin A and expand to include evaluation in rheumatoid arthritis and other auto-immune diseases. In a search for FK506 analogues, Fisons developed a 4-step screening strategy. (1) Intrinsic activity was measured in an $FK506_{bp}$ binding assay using $[^3H]$-17 propyl FK506 as the ligand. (2) Inhibition of IL-2 production in the Jurkat cell line was then measured and provided information on cell penetration as well as evidence for *in vitro* immunosuppressant activity. (3) A graft versus host (GVH) response, induced by injection of DA rat splenocytes into DA/Lewis rats, was then employed as a measure of *in vivo* immunosuppressant activity. (4) Finally, therapeutic efficacy was measured in a rat monoarticular arthritis model. FK506 and rapamycin had comparable potencies as inhibitors of binding to FK506$_{bp}$ (IC_{50} values = 300–500 pM) whereas

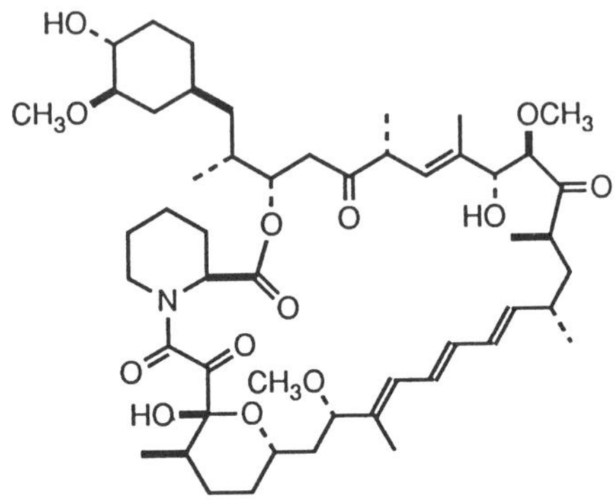

Rapamycin

cyclosporin A was inactive. FK506 was a potent inhibitor of IL-2 production (IC_{50} = 50 pM) and was approximately 100 times more potent than cyclosporin. In this system, rapamycin was much less active with only small changes in IL-2 formation observed at relatively high concentrations (10 nM). With the exception of rapamycin, there was a positive correlation between activity of FK506 analogues against IL-2 release and the GVH response. FK506 inhibited rat antigen arthritis in the same dose range as the GVH response (1–10 mg/kg p.o.) and was approximately 10 times more potent than cyclosporin. FK506 was also effective against rabbit monoarticular arthritis. Of particular interest, with respect to future clinical studies, were the observations that therapeutic dosing inhibited established arthritis in these models and that withdrawal of the drug resulted in recurrence of arthritis.

Dr. J. Y. Chang (Wyeth-Ayerst) then reviewed the pharmacology of rapamycin, another macrolide which has structural similarities with FK506. The agent was originally shown to be an effective anti-microbial agent *in vivo* in the mid-1970s [Meiser, et al.]. Interest in rapamycin was heightened when the immunosuppressive activity of FK506 was discovered. Subsequently, as described above, rapamycin was shown to bind to the $FK506_{bp}$. In a mouse thymocyte proliferation assay, rapamycin was approximately 10 times more potent than cyclosporin A (IC_{50} values = 2.8 nM and 32.9 nM, respectively). Despite sharing a common binding protein, the pharmacology of rapamycin and FK506 diverge mechanistically at the level of the T cell. In contrast to FK506, rapamycin was a poor inhibitor of IL-2 formation but studies carried out in collaboration with Dr. J. Kay (Sussex University, UK) demonstrated that rapamycin inhibited the effects of IL-2: proliferation of an IL-2 dependent pig T cell line was inhibited by rapamycin ($IC_{50} \sim 5$ pM) whereas FK506 was inactive at concentration up to 100 nM. Rapamycin has been evaluated widely in transplant models and the compound extended graft survival in models of skin, heart, kidney, bone marrow, pancreas and bowel transplantation in a range of species from rodent to primate. In general, rapamycin was less effective in extending graft survival in the higher species. Comparative data were presented in a rat skin graft model. Rapamycin was approximately 100 times more potent than cyclosporin A when dosed intraperitoneally. Combination of rapamycin and cyclosporin A in this model provided evidence for modest synergy. Anti-arthritic activity was demonstrated in the rat adjuvant model. Administering rapamycin 3 times weekly produced dose-dependent inhibition in the developing adjuvant model with an ED_{50} of 2 mg/kg, which is comparable to cyclosporin A. Rapamycin was also effective in the established adjuvant model with an ED_{50} value of approximately 4 mg/kg. More frequent dosing regimens showed similar results. In view of its encouraging pharmacological profile, clinical studies with rapamycin will commence shortly. As with FK506, the initial target will be transplantation and, prompted by the animal model synergy, combination therapy with cyclosporin A may be a possibility. Studies in rheumatic disease will depend on the safety profile obtained in the transplant trials.

From this workshop, it is clear that numerous approaches are being taken to discover and develop new drugs potentially useful in the management of chronic inflammatory diseases. Pending the successful outcome of clinical trials with these promising agents, we can look forward with optimism to having new weapons to combat these severe and persistent illness.

References

Djuric, S. W., Collins, P. W., Jones, P. H., Shone, R. L., Tsai, B. S., Fretland, D. J., Butchko, G. M., Villani-Price, D., Keith, R. H., Zemaitis, J. M., Metcalf, L. and Bauer, R. F. (1989). J. Med. Chem. 32, 6: 1145–1147.

Johnson, W. H., Roberts, N. A. and Borkakoti, N. (1987). J. Enz. Inhibition. 2: 1–22.

Kino, T., Hatanaka, H., Hashimoto, M., Nishiyama, M., Goto, T., Okuhara, M., Kohsaka, M., Aoki, H., Imanaka, H. (1987). J. Antibiotics. 40, 9: 1249–1255.

Meiser, B. M., Wang, J. and Morris, R. E. (1989). Progress in Immunology. 7: 1195–1198.

Sahoo, S. P., Graham, D. W., Acton, J., Biftu, T., Bugianesi, R. L., Girotra, N. N., Kuo, C., Ponpipom, M. M., Doebber, T. W., Wu, M. S., Hwang, S., Lam, M., MacIntyre, D. E., Bach, T. J., Luell, S., Meurer, R., Davies, P., Alberts, A. W. and Chabala, J. C. (1990). American Chemical Society National Meeting, Boston. April 1990.

Schnyder, J., Bollinger, P. and Payne, T. (1990). Agents and Actions. 30, 3/4: 350.

Siekierka, J. J., Hung, S. H. Y., Poe, M., Lin, C. S. and Sigal, N. H. (1989). Nature. 341: 755–757.

AAS 35
Progress in Inflammation
Research and Therapy

Role of Cytokines in Inflammation and Autoimmunity

J. E. Talmadge and D. R. Twardzik

University of Nebraska, Med. Ctr., Omaha, NE, USA and Oncogene, Seattle, WA, USA

Cytokines have significant potential for therapeutic utility, as well as a role in clinical disease associated with inappropriate immunologic responses. Although most cytokine-receptor interactions are a necessary part of a normal functioning immune system they also contribute to autoimmune and inflammatory disorders. However, the distinction between a specific regulatory verses an inductive role for cytokines, growth factors and eicosanoids in inflammation and autoimmunity has not yet been fully determined. Elucidation of the complexities of the cytokine cascade, their cell-surface receptors and the cellular response they invoke, during autoimmune and inflammatory disease, is only beginning and requires additional study.

Initial therapeutic strategies for these indications have focused on receptors that bind to and block autocrine and paracrine cytokine induced phenomena, as well as neutralizing antibodies to either cytokines or their receptors. Secondary strategies include those that prevent maturation or production of the cytokines such as interleukin converting enzyme inhibitors and or drugs that block production of the cytokines such as adenyl cyclase inducers which prevent the accumulation of TNF mRNA. Longer term, higher risk and more "sexy" strategies include ones that will allow the identification of the contact pharmacophore and the design of peptidomimetics with the potential to act as orally active antagonists. Clearly the ultimate goal is the design of non-peptidal mimetics with superior pharmacokinetics and oral activity.

Regardless of the developmental strategy, the critical target molecules as well as their mechanism in the clinical pathology of autoimmune disease and inflammation remains to be identified. Thus, the emphasis during the Cytokine I workshop was on: (1) the demonstration of a role for specific cytokines within models of autoimmune disease and inflammation, (2) the identification of and design of analyses for surrogates, both for disease progression and therapeutic activity and (3) the design of novel therapeutic leads and strategies.

Wim B. van den Berg of the Univ. Hospital Nijmegen, The Netherlands, with collaborators from Pfizer Central Research, Groton CT. discussed the *In Vivo Evidence For A Key Role Of IL-1 In Cartilage Destruction In Experimental Arthritis*. In these studies r Mu IL-1 was injected into the knee joint of mice. It was found that 30 and 300 but not 3 U/Animal decreased prostaglandin levels and proteoglycan synthesis. Histiological examination demonstrated a decrease in cartilage with an increase in infiltrating inflammatory cells. In other, more pharmacologic relevant, studies using antigen induced disease the injection of mBSA into the joint of sensitized animals increased the level of IL-1 which peaked at 6 hrs post injection. Neutralizating antibody demonstrated that the increase in IL-1 was largely specific for IL-1 alpha with only a slight increase in IL-1 beta. Subsequent studies demonstrated that the clinical pathology could be blocked with the injection of soluble IL-1 receptor as well as antibodies to the receptor or IL-1 alpha and beta. Control studies using neutralizing antibody to TNF demonstrated that TNF had no significant effect in the pathogenesis of this model of inflammation.

S. R. Smith of Schering Plough Research, Bloomfield, NJ. presented a discussion on the *Effects Of Recombinant IFN-g, IL-4 And IL-6 On The Development of Experimental Allergic Encephalomyelitis (EAE) In Mice*. In these studies the effect of pharmacologic levels of IL-4, IL-6 and IFN-g administered following induction of EAE was examined. The encephalitogen was injected subcutaneously into each of the hind foot pads and the cervical region and then the animals were injected intravenously with 400 ng of pertussis toxin. The injection of 5 ng of IL-4 (subcutaneously) began at the time of immunization and continued daily for 13–14 days and increased the incidence and severity of disease, while 50 ng/animal of IL-6 increased the incidence and decreased the time to disease onset, but did not increase the disease severity. The ability of the cytokines to exacerbate EAE was dependant on suboptimal induction of disease and under condition of maximal induction this additive effect was not observed. In other studies, using IFN-g, they found that the injection of 20 ng/animal/day of r Mu IFN-g delayed the onset and decreased the incidence of EAE. In partial agreement with this observation it was found that the injection of neutralizing antibodies to IFN-g increased the severity of disease but did not increase the incidence or the time of EAE onset. Follow-up studies were undertaken in which hybridoma cells, secreting either antibodies to IL-6 or IFN-g, were entrapped in alginate beads and injected into animals with EAE. In these studies animals bearing hybridoma cells producing anti IL-6 had a decreased severity of EAE; while animals with hybridoma cells producing anti IFN-g, had an increase in the severity of disease and an earlier appearance of the lesions. The most striking observation was the effect of IFN-g on clinical expression of EAE suggesting a potential clinical application for IFN-g in the treatment of CNS inflammatory diseases.

Wim B. van den Berg of the Univ. Hospital Nijmegen, The Netherlands presented their studies on the *Role Of PMN In Cartilage Destruction*. In these murine studies of antigen induced arthritis (mBSA) the loss of prelabeled proteoglycan (PG) from the patellar cartilage *in vivo* and *ex vivo* incorporation of ^{35}S-sulfate into PG was examined. The models of PMN deficiency which were used included beige mice, whose PMNs are deficient in elastase, mice irradiated with 750 rads, which results in a 98% loss of PMNs or mice injected with nitrogen mustard which results in a 90% loss of PMNs. In all cases only minor, and non-significant effects on PG loss and inhibition of PG synthesis were observed. This was in contrast to a pathologic role for PMNs that they found with immune complex (IC) induced arthritis. In normal mice IC induced arthritis results in a 57 percent degradation of cartilage whereas in neutropenic mice there was only a 10% decrease. However, the decrease in cartilage degradation did not occur in beige mice suggesting that elastase was not critical to the cartilage degradation by PMNs. It was hypothesized that IL-1 was the major induction signal in cartilage degradation and that PMNs provided an amplification of the cartilage degradation.

S. J. Foster of ICI pharmaceuticals, Merside, Alderley Park, Macclesfield, Cheshire U.K. presented a discussion on the topic *Do Leukotrines Mediate TNF-Alpha Production During Acute Inflammatory Reactions.* Based on *in vitro* studies they demonstrated that leukotrines (LT) increase IL-1 and TNF levels, while prostaglandins (PG) decrease TNF and perhaps IL-1 levels. In these *ex vivo* studies, the rat air pouch model was used to evaluate the role of selective 5-lipoxygenase (5-LO) inhibitors on TNF production induced by zymosan or LPS. They found that zymosan induced both LTB_4 and LTC_4 while LPS induced only LTB_4. The kinetics of TNF induction by LPS and zymosan also differed with peak TNF induction by LPS occurring at 2 hrs and peak levels with zymosan occurring at 4–8 hrs post stimulation. In these studies LT inhibitors decreased LT levels, but not PG or TNF levels following administration of both inducers of an inflammatory response. It was concluded that LTs are not mediators of TNF production during acute inflammation at least within the air pouch model.

M. Finch-Arietta of Hoffmann-La Roche Inc. Nutley, NJ presented studies on *Cytokine Production In Whole Blood Ex Vivo.* An assay of cytokine production from clinical samples of whole blood was developed. In this seven hour procedure, suboptimal levels of LPS are added to cultures of whole blood (250 microliter) which were primed *in vitro* with IFN-gamma. In a dose dependant manner LPS significantly increased the levels of IL-1 and TNF as assayed by an ELISA assay. This analysis strategy provides an *ex vivo* analysis of cytokine bio-synthesis that avoids non-specific monocyte activation, and may provide a surrogate for clinical trials of antiinflammatory agents, as well as, a prognostic or diagnostic indicator.

W. Galbraight of E. I. du Pont de Nemours & Co., Inc., Wilmington, DE. presented their studies on the *Effect Of IL-1 Muteins On Cartilage Degradation And As Inducers Of Acute Inflammation.* Several IL-1 mutants were cloned that differed at their N-terminus. In one such mutant where the first 2 residues (Ala-Pro) of native IL-1 were replaced with Thr-Met and Glu was substituted for Arg at position 4 a significant decrease in activity was observed compared to native IL-1 beta. This was determined using bovine nasal cartilage which was incubated with or without the muteins for 40 hrs; the media was analyzed for proteoglycan degradation and the cartilage was analyzed for proteoglycan synthesis. The proteoglycan synthesis-inhibiting activity was reduced up to 20%, and the proteoglycan-degrading activity was reduced to 2% of the activity of the native IL-1 beta. *In vivo* activity as measured by the acute induction of inflammation (paw edema) was also depressed following injection of the mutant on an equimolar basis with the native IL-1 beta. However, if higher doses of the mutant protein were injected equal levels of activity could be induced. It appears that the positive charge at position 4 (Arg) may be important for the activity of IL-1 beta. Although, position 4 may be part of the contact surface between IL-1 and the receptor, it was suggested that it is more likely to be responsible for maintaining a preferred confirmation for receptor binding.

P. E. Poubelle of CHUS, Sharbrooke, Canada, with collaborators from CEN-Sacity, France presented their studies on the observation that *Leukotriene B4 Up-Regulates IL-6 Rather Than IL-1 Synthesis In Human Monocytes.* The effect of LTB_4 on IL-1/IL-6 protein levels and mRNA accumulation by normal blood monocytes was reported. LTB_4 induced IL-6, but not IL-1, protein release and mRNA accumulation. The optimal dose of LTB_4 was 10^{-8} M LTB_4 with a significant threshold of activity at 10^{-10} M. It was cautioned that an artifactual conclusion could be reached if a bioassay is utilized in which both IL-6 and IL-1 are active, such as the thymocyte proliferation assay. Appropriate immunoassays suggested that LTB_4 could simultaneously down regulate IL-1 production by monocytes, however, this could be mediated through IL-6 since it has recently been reported to partially inhibit IL-1 generation (1).

E. C. Arner of E. I. du Pont de Nemours & Co., Inc., Wilmington, DE presented their studies on the *Modulation Of Interleukin-1-Induced Alterations In Cartilage Proteoglycan Metabolism By Activation Of Protein Kinase C.* IL-1 acts through a receptor mediated process, although the mechanism of signal transduction is unclear. Because protein kinase C (PKC) is known to play a role in biological processes and was recently suggested to regulate plasminogen activator production by synovial cells and collagenase production by chondrocytes, PKC inducers and inhibitors were evaluated to determine if PKC had a regulatory role on IL-1 induced cartilage degradation. In these studies PKC agonists alone had no effect on proteoglycan (PG) metabolism, although they inhibited the stimulation of PG degradation and inhibition of PG synthesis induced by IL-1. This biological activity could be blocked by the PKC antagonist Staurosporin. In separate studies the PKC agonist mezerein alone increased PGE_2 release from cartilage and synergized with IL-1 in stimulating PGE_2 release. This differential effect of PKC agonists on IL-1 induced activities (PG metabolism and PGE_2) suggested that these processes are independently regulated at the post receptor level. They suggested that the IL-1 effect on PG degradation is not mediated via PKC, although PKC may have a regulatory role in IL-1 induced cartilage destruction.

T. Matter of Johaes Gutenberg University, Mainz, FRG and collaborators from RUSH Medical College, Chicago, IL presented their studies on *Leflunomide, An Immunomodulator With Antiproliferative Properties, Inhibits EGF-Receptor Tyrosine Kinase*. The active metabolite of Leflunomide, a drug designed for therapeutic activity in autoimmune disease, has antiproliferative activity for all cell types tested. However, the IC-50 varied among cells of different origins and was not species specific. It was suggested that a common mechanism, central to cell division, might be disrupted by this drug. The effect of the active metabolite was examined on EGF-receptor tyrosine specific kinase activity, as an example of growth factor dependant tyrosine kinase activity. Multiple analyses demonstrated that a significant decrease in phosphokinase activity occurred at a concentration of analogue sufficient to inhibit 50% of cellular proliferation. Thus, the hypothesis was suggested that the mechanism of Leflunomide activity may be the inhibition of a cytokine specific tyrosine kinase. This inhibition occurred with IL-3, 4, 5 and 6 but not IL-1. A slight effect was observed on IL-2. In addition no effect of IFN-g was observed, although a potent activity on CSF-m and CSF-gm activity was reported.

In summary, supportive evidence for a role of several cytokines in the pathogenesis of autoimmunity and inflammation was demonstrated in animal models. In several incidences a specific hierarchy of activity was suggested and an assay using whole blood was developed for therapeutic surrogates to be used in clinical protocols.

Preliminary immunoregulatory roles for specific cytokines and eicosanoids were suggested, including the immunotherapeutic activity for IFN-gamma as well as the therapeutic potential of a tyrosine kinase inhibitor.

References

Schindler, R., Mancilla, J., Endres, S., Ghorbani, R., Clark, S. C. and Dinarello, C. A. (1990). Correlations and interactions in the production of Interleukin-6 (IL-6), IL-1, and tumor necrosis factor (TNF) in human mononuclear cells: IL-6 suppresses IL-1 and TNF. Blood. 75: 40–47.

AAS 35
Progress in Inflammation
Research and Therapy

Adhesion Proteins: In vitro and In vivo Studies of Leukocyte-endothelial Interactions

L. G. Letts and D. Y. Liu***

*Boehringer Ingelheim Pharmaceuticals, Ridgefield, Connecticut, USA and
**Cetus Corporation, Emeryville, California 94608, USA

Adhesion of leukocytes to endothelials cells is a critical step for host defense as well as the progression of an inflammatory response. The inhibition of the process of cell activation and recognition, which requires cell-cell contact and if left unchecked can result in pathophysiological complications, provides a novel means of therapeutic intervention. The events leading to leukocyte adhesion and emigration from the vasculature as a result of immune-mediated and inflammatory stimuli have therefore been the focus of an explosion of attention within the biotechnology and pharmaceutical industries as well as academe. An indication of this is the workshop on adhesion proteins at the 5th International Conference of the Inflammation Research Association. Only two years ago at the last conference, there was no single workshop devoted to adhesion. This year, there were ten presentations ranging from *in vitro* studies describing mechanisms of adhesion or utilizing carbohydrates and vasoactive neuropeptides as cellular adhesion inhibitors to the demonstration of *in vivo* efficacy of several monoclonal antibodies directed against membrane adhesion molecules in animal models of inflammatory diseases. This summary will attempt to outline the significant findings of the studies presented at the workshop and to convey a sense of the future in this area of investigation as discussed by the participants and audience.

A major presentation was made by C. Wayne Smith of Baylor College of Medicine for the purpose of summarizing the recent efforts of his laboratory in studying the characteristics of CD_{18}-

dependent and -independent mechanisms of neutrophil adhesion and emigration through the endothelium. It appears that the adhesion molecule, murine MEL-14 or the human LAM-1, has an important role in mediating the adherence of leukocytes to endothelial cells distinct from its originally described function as the lymphocyte homing receptor. As a member of the LEC-CAM family of proteins it has the unique qualities of being expressed on neutrophils and monocytes and downregulated as a result of cell activation by chemotactic factors, such as C5a and FMLP. Data was presented which demonstrates that LAM-1 is involved in CD_{18}-independent mechanisms of neutrophil adhesion. This resulted from the use of LAM-1 monoclonal antibodies and neutrophils form LAD (Leukocyte Adhesion Deficiency) individuals. Although ELAM-1 has also been shown to participate in CD_{18}- independent mechanisms, it is not known whether LAM-1 and ELAM-4 form an adhesion ligand pair.

In a related presentation (one of three *in vitro* studies) Cheng-Po Sung from SmithKline Beecham Pharmaceuticals described his efforts in studying the involvement of carbohydrates in the adhesion of leukocytes to endothelial cells. Members of the LEC-CAM family of adhesion protein (LAM-1, ELAM-1, VCAM) are characterized by their lectin-like structure. Using a monocytic cell line, U-937, as a model system Sung showed that fucose 1-P, fucoidin, lactose 1-P and fructose 1-P all inhibited the binding of U-937 cells to TNF-α-stimulated human umbilical vein endothelial cells. The adhesion binding molecule for the inhibitory carbohydrates has not yet been identified. The second presentation in the "*in vitro*" phase of this workshop was made by William Fleming of the Upjohn Company. The binding of functional subpopulations of T lymphocytes was studied resulting in two interesting findings. One was that CD45RA "suppressor-inducer/naive" cells upon activation by IL-2 or IL-4 exhibit increased levels of CD29 which defines the subset of "helper-inducer/memory" cells. Furthermore, IL-2 stimulated T cells (naive or memory) adhere better than unstimulated cells to IL-1β-activated endothelial cells or IFN-gamma-activated synovial fibroblasts. This suggests some common mechanisms whereby memory T cells become trapped in the rheumatoid synovium. Finally, the last study in this section was presented by M.D. Josephs of Georgetown University Medical Center. Angiopeptin, a somatostatin-like octapeptide,

Table I. Effect of Antibodies of Adhesion Molecules on Animal Models of Inflammation

Antibody to Adhesion	*Animal Model of Disease*	*Investigation*
CD_{18}	Indomethacin-induced ulcer in rabbit	Wallace, U. of Calgary
CD_{18}	PMA-induced cell and plasma leakage in rabbit lung	Meurer, Merck
CD_{18}	Antigen-induced airway hyper-responsiveness in guinea pigs	Noonan, Boehringer Ingelheim
CD_{18}	Endotoxin shock in rabbit	Weldon, Boehringer Ingelheim
ICAM-1	Schwartzman-like lesions in rabbit	Argenbright, Boehringer Ingelheim
ELAM-1	Antigen-induced airway hyper-responsiveness in monkeys	Wegner, Boehringer Ingelheim

was found to be inhibitory for the adherence of rat spleen cells to coronary arterial endothelial cells. The data suggest that inhibition is mediated by protein kinase A acting through adenylate cyclase activity.

The *in vivo* effects of specific antibodies directed towards either the beta subunit of the CD_{11}/CD_{18} complex, ICAM-1 or ELAM-1 adhesion proteins in various inflammation models were described in another six presentations.

John Wallace (Calgary) showed that in a rabbit model of NSAID-induced gastropathy, the anti-CD18 antibody IB-4 prevented leucocyte margination and reduced the extent of the hemorrhagic damage. The reduction was greater than 85% and further supported his findings in earlier studies (neutrophil depleted animals) of the role of the neutrophil in NSAID-gastropathy. The same antibody was shown by R. Meurer and colleagues (Merck Sharp & Dohme) to significantly inhibit the accumulation and extravasation of plasma from the lungs of rabbits when injected intravenously with PMA. Interestingly, pretreatment with IB-4 (same animals) did not inhibit the systemic reduction of circulating leukocytes or neutrophils subsequent to the administration of PMA. Steven Weldon and colleagues (Boehringer Ingelheim Pharmaceuticals) showed that $R_{15,7}$ (another anti-CD_{18} antibody) in a rabbit model of endotoxin shock protected against the severe hypotension and death which was seen with control (mouse IgG) treated animals. He reported that in the anti-CD_{18} treated animals peripheral neutrophil counts remained significantly higher and indicated the importance of the neutrophil in this form of shock.

L. Argenbright (Boehringer Ingelheim) presented data in a rabbit shwartzman-like model that the extravasation and hemorrhage was dependent upon a ICAM-1/CD_{18} interaction. He showed in an elegant fashion that either a single injection of anti-ICAM (R6.5) prior to the intradermal administration of endotoxin or a single injection of anti-ICAM prior to zymosan "challenge" was sufficient to completely inhibit the response. Further, he showed that injection of the anti-CD_{18} antibody immediately prior to the "challenge" also totally blocked the response. He illustrated that the initial intradermal injection of endotoxin primarily increased the expression of ICAM-1 on the endothelial cell surface and that "challenge" with zymosan increased the expression of a corresponding ligand on the neutrophil cell surface.

In two other studies from the Boehringer Ingelheim group, Tom Noonan reported the beneficial actions of an anti-CD_{18} antibody in antigen-induced airway hyperresponsiveness in guinea pigs. He showed that 24 hours after ovalbumin challenge to sensitized animals there was a significant increase in the BAL of neutrophils and eosinophils. In addition, a significant increase in the airway responsiveness to intravenous acetylcholine and serotonin was measurable. Pretreatment with the anti-CD_{18} antibody decreased both the cell influx into the lungs (BAL counts) and responsiveness. Craig Wegner showed that in a repeated antigen inhalation model of airway inflammation and hyperresponsiveness in monkeys, treatment with an anti-ELAM antibody (CL2) did not exhibit any effect. This was in contrast to their earlier work in which they showed that anti-ICAM-1 was effective in reducing the influx of eosinophils, airway inflammation and induction of airway hyperresponsiveness.

In summary, this workshop gained considerable attention and illustrated how rapidly this new and exciting discipline of science hasprogressed. It was clear at the conclusion of this session that the identification of adhesion proteins and the development of specific monoclonal antibodies presents a new frontier for the academician as well as the industrial scientist.

Progress in Inflammation
Research and Therapy

Cytokines and Drugs Workshop

J. T. Hom and P. L. Simon***

*Lilly Research Laboratories, Indianapolis, IN 46285, USA
**CIBA-GEIGY Pharmaceuticals Division, Summit, NJ 07901, USA

Cytokines such as IL-1, TNF and gamma-IFN are considered important mediators of inflammation and joint destruction in rheumatoid arthritis (RA). It is believed that either excessive production of these cytokines and/or insufficient synthesis of cytokine inhibitors may contribute to the pathogenesis of various inflammatory and arthritic diseases. Numerous *in vitro* as well as *in vivo* studies have provided evidence supporting the pro-inflammatory properties of IL-1. Therefore, agents which are capable of suppressing either the production of IL-1 or the various inflammatory events induced by IL-1 may be useful for the treatment of RA as well as other arthritic diseases. Various *in vivo* systems that were developed to detect such agents were addressed in the "Drugs and Cytokines" workshop. The abstracts which were presented in this workshop dealt with two major topics: (1) the ability of various drugs to inhibit the inflammatory activities induced by IL-1 and (2) the effects of drugs on the synthesis of IL-1.

With regard to the first topic, in the studies of E. O'Byrne (Ciba-Geigy, USA) inflammation and cartilage destruction were induced by three daily intra-articular injections of recombinant human interleukin-1 (rIL-1) (100 ng/injection) into knee joints of rabbits. The results of these studies demonstrated that drugs such as triamcinolone, dexamethasone, and indomethacin were effective in significantly inhibiting the influx of inflammatory cells and the production of PGE_2 and substance P, while having no effect on proteoglycan loss. Likewise, S. Chandrasekhar (Lilly Research Laboratories, USA) reported that 3 intra-articular injections of rIL-1

(30 μg/injection) into the knee joints of rats can also lead to edema, synovitis, fibroblast proliferation, and cartilage destruction as determined by histologic analyses. Moreover, these studies showed that certain drugs such as azathioprine, diclofenac, and methotrexate only reduced the soft tissue swelling induced by IL-1, whereas dexamethasone and various NSAIDs were found to inhibit both the swelling and cartilage/bone damage. The third paper presented by J. Hom (Lilly Research Laboratories) demonstrated that treatments with IL-1 can accelerate the development of type II collagen-induced arthritis (CIA) in mice and rats. Further studies also indicated that a variety of drugs which included steroids, NSAIDs, immunosuppressants and methotrexate could inhibit the IL-1 mediated acceleration of CIA. However, in this model mice appeared less sensitive than rats to the effects of NSAIDs. During the discussion of these presentations it was pointed out that the amount of IL-1 required for the rat model (Chandrasekhar) was considerably more than that employed in the rabbit model (O'Byrne). The possibility was raised that species variation and differences in the methods employed for evaluating the inflammatory disease can account for the difference in amount of IL-1 needed for the induction of arthritis. It was also noted that proteoglycan synthesis, a parameter employed by E. O'Byrne in her rabbit studies, appears to be fairly sensitive to the inhibitory effects of IL-1. The possibility that endotoxin contamination within the IL-1 preparation may be responsible for the inflammatory response occurring in the rats was ruled out by the following studies: (1) the level of endotoxin was determined to be within the range of 0.3–3 ng/mg of IL-1, and at the highest concentration of IL-1 injected the maximum endotoxin given would have been 0.3 ng which was not sufficient to cause histopathological changes, and (2) the ability of polymyxin B treated preparation of IL-1 to induce arthritic lesions in rats was similar to that of non-polymyxin B treated IL-1. The apparent discrepancies of the results between the studies of S. Chandrasekhar and the studies of E. O'Byrne regarding NSAID protection of IL-1 induced cartilage degradation may be due to the fact that in O'Byrne's studies cartilage degradation was evaluated by measuring proteoglycan loss, whereas, in S. Chandrasekhar's work, histologic analyses were performed. The question was raised as to why there is a need to develop IL-1 inhibitors if

NSAIDs are effective in preventing the inflammation and joint damage induced by IL-1. In response, it was proposed that the beneficial effects of NSAIDs are most likely due to their ability to prevent the occurrence of early events such as edema and influx of inflammatory cells. On the other hand, IL-1 inhibitors can potentially intervene at both the early as well as late stage of the disease in which cartilage/bone destructions represent late events.

The drug discovery efforts of many pharmaceutical companies have been designed to discover novel therapeutic agents that have as their major mechanism of action the inhibition of the production of one or more of the proinflammatory cytokines such as IL-1 or TNF. In some cases cytokine production inhibition has been discovered after the fact for a drug under development. Regardless of the mode of discovery, the claims made for cytokine production inhibition supported by *in vitro* studies need to be validated *in vivo*. In addition, it may be more useful to screen for novel agents using *in vivo* assays, which are not subject to the well known problems associated with the interpretation of *in vitro* inhibition assays. Two presentations were made on the use of animal models to examine the inhibition of cytokine production by drugs. The first of these was on the use of a model of zymosan-induced peritonitis in mice, presented by Kathleen Gans-Brangs (E. I. du Pont, USA). This model allows for the study of the sequential production of eicosanoids, cellular infiltrates, and cytokines in the peritoneal cavities of mice undergoing an acute response to an inflammatory agent. Using this model, the group at du Pont evaluated three agents reported to inhibit the production of IL-1: dexamethasone, SK&F 86002 (a dual cyclooxygenase/5-lipoxygenase inhibitor), and Tenidap (from Pfizer, a predominantly cyclooxygenase inhibitor with some weak activity towards 5-LO). As expected, dexamethasone was the most potent inhibitor of IL-1 production, in keeping with its well established antiinflammatory profile. SK&F 86002 was able to inhibit production by 75% when given at 300 mg/kg. Interestingly, although this drug was withdrawn from development due to a variety of acute and chronic toxicities, none were seen in the zymosan-induced peritonitis model at the very high doses used. However it should be pointed out that the time course of the experiment was relatively short. Tenidap failed to inhibit IL-1 production. One point which requires further investigation before this model can gain acceptance as a means for identification of drugs that can inhibit cytokine production is the question of whether the action of the drugs was indirectly mediated by the blockade of cellular infiltration, or was a direct effect on cytokine transcription, translation, processing, or secretion. This later issue was dealt with in the final presentation given by L. S. Noel, who talked about the effects of antiinflammatory drugs on the expression of IL-1 beta mRNA levels found in ankle tissues of arthritic Lewis rats (induced by group A streptococcal cell wall). Dexamethasone (0.5 mg/kg) reduced both joint swelling and levels of IL-1 beta mRNA, whereas indomethacin (2–10 mg/kg) reduced only joint swelling but had no effect on IL-1 message levels. It will be interesting to see how other drugs reported to inhibit cytokine production fair in this model.

Overall, we believe that progress is being made in developing animal models that can be used to discover novel agents that block the production or action of inflammatory cytokines such as IL-1. We still need to resolve the interpretation of experiments in which exceedingly high doses of IL-1 are used to induce a pathological change. In the future we will need to develop and implement animal models that can clearly discriminate IL-1 inhibitors from NSAIDs, a feature that many of the current models lack. Furthermore, with the recent emergence of specific IL-1 inhibitors in the form of soluble IL-1 receptor protein or the recently discovered IL-1 receptor antagonist, we have the opportunity to validate the IL-1 dependence of the models at hand, and thus make rational decisions concerning the choice of a model for drug discovery.

AAS 35
Progress in Inflammation
Research and Therapy

Therapeutic Approaches to Reduce Airway Inflammation

M. O'Donnell and A. N. Payne***

*Hoffmann-La Roche Inc., Nutley, NJ 07110, USA
**Wellcome Research Laboratories, Beckenham, England

Asthma is a chronic inflammatory disease characterized by reversible airway obstruction and bronchial hyperreactivity. Over the past few years, therapy has shifted away from an emphasis on agents to treat the spasmogenic aberration of smooth muscle to approaches directed at addressing the chronic inflammatory aspects of the disease. In connection with this, the pulmonary disease workshop focused on new therapeutic approaches to reduce pulmonary inflammation associated with asthma. Two presentations in the session described the developmental status of the chemically distinct 5-lipoxygenase inhibitors: Abbott's A-64077 and Boehringer Ingelheim's BI-L-239. The other talks concerned animal models which investigated bronchial hyperreactivity and lung inflammation, the role of IL-5 in the recruitment and activation of eosinophils, and the activation of leukocytes by platelets in response to antigen challenge. The session ended with a mini-review of the role of adhesion molecules in lung inflammation and a discussion of the potential usefulness of ICAM-1 antagonists in asthma.

The pathognomonic feature of asthma is non-specific bronchial hyperreactivity. This phenomenon has been linked to airway inflammation [1]. Many different experimental models of bronchial hyperreactivity have been developed in which the pathophysiologic role of various cell types (neutrophils, eosinophils, platelets, lymphocytes) has been investigated. Dr. D. Vincent (Institute Pasteur & Hospital Rothschild, Paris, France) described a model in anesthetized guinea-pigs in which the intratracheal administration of *E. Coli* endotoxin (LPS) elicited bronchial hyperreactivity to intravenous serotonin. The bronchial hyperreactivity induced by LPS was platelet- but not leukocyte-dependent. Dr. Vincent presented data from a subsequent series of experiments which suggested that there was a dissociation between LPS-induced bronchial hyperreactivity and airway inflammation. Various receptor antagonists and inhibitors were used to modulate LPS-induced bronchial hyperreactivity and lung inflammation, to determine whether bronchial hyperreactivity depended on increased alveolo-capillary permeability. After intratracheal administration of LPS (0.1–1 mg), the increased alveolo-capillary permeability was evaluated according to the rate of appearance of radiolabelled albumin (given intratracheally) in the blood and lung inflammation was assessed three hours later by counting the cells in bronchoalveolar lavage (BAL) fluid. The anti-histamine, mepyramine, blocked the LPS-induced increase in alveolo-capillary permeability, as did the PAF antagonist WEB 2170, whereas aspirin was ineffective. In contrast to the inhibitory effects of mepyramine and WEB 2170 on LPS-induced alveolo-capillary permeability, neither of these agents reduced the pulmonary recruitment of neutrophils induced by LPS, nor did they inhibit LPS-induced bronchial hyperreactivity. Dr. Vincent concluded that the alveolo-capillary permeability and bronchial hyperreactivity induced by the LPS resulted from separate mechanisms. LPS-induced alveolo-capillary permeability is accounted for by the presence of histamine and/or PAF, but does not contribute to bronchial hyperreactivity or recruitment of neutrophils to the airways.

Over the decades, clinical observations suggest an important association between eosinophils and asthma. For example, the degree of peripheral blood eosinophilia has been shown to correlate with the severity of airway obstruction [2, 3]. Eosinophils are increased in sputum of asthmatics, and airway histopathology indicates eosinophilic infiltration. Furthermore, with resolution of asthma severity, eosinophil numbers decrease. Recent evidence shows that instillation of antigen in the airway attracts large numbers of eosinophils, which when activated, release granular proteins. Infiltrating, activated eosinophils, through the action of cytoxic mediators may promote the development of airway inflammation by damaging airway epithelium and contracting airway smooth muscle [4, 5]. Many factors are hypothesized to participate in the recruitment and activation of eosinophils in asthma. Using a monoclonal antibody to IL-5 that was secreted by hybridoma TRFK-5 cells, Dr. R. Egan (Schering-Plough) investigated the theory that IL-5 is necessary for the recruitment and activation of eosinophils during antigen-induced anaphylaxis in guinea pigs. Eosinophil accumulation in lung tissue and BAL fluid was measured 24 hours after ovalbumin challenge (0.25% exposure for six seconds). This challenge protocol produced prolonged eosinophil-rich (6- to 10-fold increase) inflammatory leukocyte infiltration into the lungs of guinea pigs peaking at 24 hours after antigen provocation [6]. Murine anti-IL-5 administered either acutely (1–1000 μg intravenously, two hours before ovalbumin challenge) or chronically (TRFK-5 cells in alginate gel, injected into the peritoneal cavity and releasing antibody *in situ* over a four day period) produced a dose-dependent inhibition of eosinophil accumulation with an ID_{50} value of approximately 10 μg. Neither denatured nor isotype control antibodies, at doses as high as 10 mg, attenuated eosinophil infiltration. These studies indicate that IL-5 is necessary for eosinophil infiltration into the lungs of allergic guinea pigs and suggest that anti-IL-5 agents could be useful for treating pulmonary inflammation. Unfortunately, it is impossible to use this monoclonal antibody approach to examine the role of eosinophils in bronchial hyperreactivity in this particular model of antigen-induced anaphylaxis since bronchial hyperreactivity is not evident.

Leukotrienes (LTs) are a family of bioactive lipids that result from the metabolism of arachidonic acid by 5-lipoxygenase. The peptidoleukotrienes LTC_4, LTD_4, and LTE_4 have a variety of pharmacologic effects on respiratory, cardiovascular, and gastrointestinal systems [7, 8]. They produce smooth muscle contraction, cause myocardial depression, increase vascular permeability, enhance mucus production, decrease mucociliary transport, attract leukocytes to sites of cellular injury, and stimulate leukocyte activation. These properties, and the detection of LTs in effected tissue and biological fluids suggest that LTs play a significant role in a number of allergic and inflammatory diseases including asthma, adult respiratory distress syndrome, septic shock, myocardial ischemia, psoriasis, inflammatory bowel disease, and arthritis. For these reasons, the idea of inhibiting the 5-lipoxygenase enzyme is considered an attractive target for discovering novel agents to treat inflammatory disease states in man.

In the workshop, two chemically distinct 5-lipoxygenase inhibitors were described; one orally-active (A-64077) and one aerosol-active (BI-L-239).

Dr. C. Lanni (Abbott) briefly highlighted the two clinical studies which have been completed in asthmatics with A-64077 (zileuton). The effect of oral A-64077 on the early and late asthmatic response to inhaled allergen was studied in mild atopic asthmatics in a randomized, double-blind, placebo-controlled, cross-over study [9]. Of the nine male asthmatics who completed the study, all had a dual response to inhaled allergen (house dust mite or mixed grass pollen). Subjects ingested a single dose of A-64077 (800 mg) or matching placebo and allergen challenge was performed three hours later. A-64077 reduced urinary LTE_4 excretion (an index of *in vivo* LT production) by 50%. At the dose used in this study, A-64077 had no significant inhibiting effect on airway responses to allergen. However, this may be due to inadequate inhibition of 5-lipoxygenase at the single 800 mg dose used.

Dr. Lanni also reported on the *in vivo* and *ex vivo* effects of pretreatment with A-64077 in 13 asthmatics following cold-dry air-induced hyperventilation [10]. Subjects received a single oral 800 mg dose of A-64077 or placebo in a randomized, double blind, placebo controlled, crossover design. Airway response to cold-dry air hyperventilation was assessed three hours after drug administration. Baseline FEV_1 was unchanged after receiving A-64077. There was a significant inhibition (48%) of the bronchospastic response to cold-dry air hyperventilation with A-64077 compared to placebo. Whole blood, drawn prior to drug administration and just prior to assessment of airway response, was challenged with calcium ionophore, A23187. The plasma was chromatographed and assayed for immunoreactive LTB_4 and TXB_2. There was a 70% reduction in ionophore-challenged plasma levels of LTB_4 whereas TXB_2 production was unaffected. These data suggest that the 5-lipoxygenase derivatives of arachidonic acid may play a significant role in mediating cold-air induced bronchoconstriction.

Dr. C. Wegner (Boehringer Ingelheim) described the *in vivo* pharmacological profile of the selective 5-lipoxygenase inhibitor,

BI-L-239, in two animal models of asthma. In anesthetized cynomolgus monkeys, inhaled BI-L-239 provided a dose-dependent inhibition of the inhaled *Ascaris*-induced acute LTC_4 release (maximum inhibition $73 \pm 12\%$), late phase bronchoconstriction (maximum inhibition $41 \pm 3\%$) and neutrophil infiltration (maximum inhibition $63 \pm 16\%$). In conscious sheep, inhaled BI-L-239 provided a dose-dependent inhibition of the inhaled *Ascaris*-induced late phase bronchoconstriction (maximum inhibition 66%), eosinophil/neutrophil infiltration (maximum inhibition 61%) and increased airway responsiveness (maximum inhibition 82%). The acute bronchoconstriction was not inhibited in either species. The Boehringer-Ingelheim compound is currently undergoing aerosolized toxicological evaluation in preparation for eventual clinical study.

Dr. R. H. Gundel (Boehringer) described the release of bronchoactive mediators into the airways of allergic primates during the acute response to specific antigen inhalation. In 12 *Ascaris suum* sensitive cynomolgus monkeys, respiratory system resistance was measured prior to and after antigen inhalation. Bronchoalveolar lavage was then performed. Immunoreactive LTC_4, prostaglandin D_2 (PGD_2) and histamine were quantitated in BAL samples. LTC_4 increased 40-fold, PGD_2 increased 10-fold, and histamine increased 20-fold in the BAL samples collected after *Ascaris* challenge. Increases in LTC_4, PGD_2, and histamine levels were inhibited 71%, 51%, and 43%, respectively, by dexamethasone (1 mg/kg, p.o., 1, 4 and 24 hr pretreatment). The increase in pulmonary resistance was not inhibited by dexamethasone. Surprisingly, the PAF receptor antagonist, WEB 2170 (3 mg/kg, p.o.), blocked the generation and release of leukotrienes and prostaglandins.

A role for platelets in inflammation has gained considerable support in light of the demonstration that platelets bear low affinity IgE receptors which respond to antigen stimulation [11]. Furthermore, platelets accumulate within the pulmonary vasculature in many animal species and in man following antigen challenge or the administration of inflammatory mediators (e.g., PAF) [12, 13]. Dr. Vargaftig and co-workers (Unitè Associèe Institut Pasteur-Inserm, Paris, France) investigated whether platelets obtained from actively sensitized guinea-pigs and transferred to non-immunized animals retain the ability to recognize antibody. Washed platelets, from actively sensitized guinea pigs, were transfused into non-sensitized guinea pigs. Subsequent administration of intravenous antigen induced marked, long-lasting leukopenia (approximately 50% at 60 minutes), but no thrombocytopenia [14]. This suggests that platelets release a material which activates leukocytes. However, release of this material was secretion independent since no platelet aggregation or ATP or serotonin release accompanied the leukopenia. Indomethacin (10 mg/kg, i.v.) enhanced and nedocromil sodium (100 mg/kg, i.v.) or the mixed cyclooxygenase (CO)/lipoxygenase (LO) inhibitor, BW 755C (10 mg/kg, i.v.), inhibited the leukopenia. Leukopenia was unaffected by the PAF antagonist, WEB 2170, and the selective LO inhibitor, BW A4C (50 mg/kg, i.v.), suggesting that neither PAF nor LO derivatives are involved and that BW 755C may operate via free radical scavenging. Cetirizine (10–30 mg/kg, i.v.), an anti-histamine which blocks eosinophil migration and platelet cytotoxicity, inhibited the leukopenia; however, other anti-histamines (e.g., terfenadine and mepyramine) were inactive. Nedocromil sodium and cetirizine may operate by a mechanism similar to inhibition of *in vitro* cytotoxicity or on the endothelium. During the discussion period, Dr. G. Letts commented that his laboratory repeated these experiments and confirmed these *in vivo* findings. It is also noteworthy that the leukopenia was completely prevented by heparin (100 U/ml). In conclusion, Dr. Vargaftig suggested that interference with this platelet-leukocyte interaction may be a promising target for rational drug design by virtue of its specificity.

The interaction of leukocyte adhesion molecules with their respective ligands on other cells and on the extracellular matrix is now recognized to be a key process in cellular localization and migration, such as that occuring in diapedesis. This interplay of adhesion proteins and their ligands is also important in cell-cell communication, signalling, and the interaction of cytotoxic T-cells with their targets in host defense reactions [15]. Currently, there is considerable interest in the role of adhesion molecules in lung inflammation and in particular, asthma. Reflecting this interest, in his second presentation, Dr. C. Wegner (Boehringer Ingelheim) gave a highly informative mini-review on this subject. In order for leukocytes to migrate into inflamed tissue, they must first adhere to the microvascular endothelium. This process is controlled by the interaction of leukocyte adhesion molecules such as the integrins LFA-1 and Mac-1, and the selectin, Mel-14, with ligands on the endothelial cell (e.g., ICAM-1, intercellular adhesion molecule-1; ELAM-1, endothelial leukocyte adhesion molecule-1; and GMP-140, granule membrane protein-140) which can be rapidly upregulated by inflammatory cytokines (e.g., IL-1, TNFα). Once through the endothelial layer, VLA-1, -2, and -3 are extracellular matrix adhesion proteins which can interact with laminin, collagen and fibronectin. VLA-4 functions as both a matrix and cell receptor, in the latter respect binding to a molecule termed VCAM-1 (vascular cell adhesion molecule-1), a member of the immunoglobulin superfamily. On activation of the leukocyte, Mel-14 is shed allowing the leukocyte to marginate into the extravascular space and migrate thereafter under the control of matrix adhesion molecule interactions (e.g., VLA-1 and laminin/collagen) to the site of the inflammatory lesion.

Dr. Wegner went on to describe the results from a recent study [16] in which he and his group investigated the possible contribution of ICAM-1 to the pathogenesis of antigen-induced eosinophil migration and bronchial hyperreactivity in cynomologous monkeys. In these animals, ICAM-1 is expressed on both the bronchial vascular endothelium and airway epithelium following chronic antigen inhalation. Three alternate-day inhalations of *Ascaris* extract antigen induced a consistent increase in bronchial hyperreactivity (8-fold) as assessed with inhaled methacholine and a marked eosinophilia which was assayed by bronchoalveolar lavage. Airway eosinophilia was markedly attenuated (60%) and bronchial hyperreactivity was nearly abolished by intravenous pretreatment with a mouse anti-human ICAM-1 monoclonal antibody (R6.5; 1.76 mg/kg daily). Comparable results were obtained in four out of six animals when the antibody was given by inhalation. While the effect of the ICAM-1 monoclonal antibody on bronchial hyperreactivity may be due to attenuation of eosinophil migration, antagonism of an ICAM-1 dependent interaction of eosinophils with the airway epithelium may also be important. In contrast to these positive results with a monoclonal antibody to ICAM-1, similar experiments with a murine anti-human ELAM-1 monoclonal antibody (CL-2) failed to demonstrate a role for ELAM-1 in either antigen-induced eosinophil infiltration or bronchial hyperreactivity.

Dr. Wegner's talk provoked much discussion, illustrating the topical nature of this subject. A central issue regarding possible clinical applications is the ability to obtain selective inhibition of inflammatory adhesion mechanisms without compromising host defense reactions.

In summary, it is a challenge to develop novel, biologically-active compounds to treat the inflammatory component of asthma. This workshop reviewed the recent progress in the preclinical and clinical development of two selective 5-lipoxygenase inhibitors (A-64077 and BI-L-239) and explored some promising new targets for rational drug discovery. Antagonists of ICAM-1, IL-5 and platelet-leukocyte interactions were identified as novel therapeutic approaches to reduce airway inflammation and bronchial hyperreactivity associated with asthma.

References

Holgate, S. T., Beesley R. and Twentyman, O. P. (1987). Clin. Sci. 73: 561–572.
Horn, B. R., Robin, E. D., Theodore, J. and Van Kessel, A. (1975). New Engl. J. Med. 292: 1152–1155.
Burrows, B., Hasan, F. M., Barbee, R. A., Halonen, M. and Lebowitz, M. (1980). Am. Rev. Respir. Dis. 122: 709–719.
Wardlaw, A. J., Dunnette, S., Gleich, G. J., Collins, J. V. and Kay, B. A. (1988). Am. Rev. Respir. Dis. 137: 62–69.
Frigas, E. and Gleich, G. J. (1986). J. Allergy Clin. Immunol. 77: 527–537.
Gulbenkian, A. R., Fernandez, X., Kreutner, W., Minnicozzi, M., Watnick, A. S., Kung, T. and Egan, R. W. (1990). Am. Rev. Respir. Dis. 142: 680–685.
Drazen, J. M. and Austen, K. F. (1987). Am. Rev. Respir. Dis. 136: 985–998.
Piper, P. J. (1989). Arzneimittel-Forschung. 39: 1005–1008.
Hui, K. P., Taylor I. K. and Barnes, P. J. (1990). Am. Rev. Respir. Dis. 141: A32.
Israel, E., Dermarkian, R. M., Rosenberg, M. A., Rubin, P. and Drazen, J. M. (1990). Am. Rev. Respir. Dis. 141: A175.
Joseph, M., Capron, A., Ameisen, J. C., Vorng, H., Pancre, V., Kusnierz, J. P. and Aurialt, C. (1986). Eur. J. Immunol. 16: 306–312.
Lellouch-Tubiana, A., Lefort, J., Simon, M.-T., Pfister, A. and Vargaftig, B. B. (1988). Am. Rev. Respir. Dis. 137: 948–954.
Knauer, K. A., Lichtenstein, L. M., Adkinson, N. K. and Fish, J. E. (1981). N. Engl. J. Med. 304: 1404–1407.
Pretolani, M., Random, J. and Vargaftig, B. B. (1990). Br. J. Pharmacol. 100: 185–189.
Springer, T. A. (1990). Nature. 346: 425–434.
Wegner, C. D., Gundel, R. H., Reilly, P., Haynes, N., Letts, L. G. and Rothlein, R. (1990). Science. 247: 456–459.

AAS 35
Progress in Inflammation
Research and Therapy

Osteoarthritis

E. R. Schwartz and R. L. Goldberg***

*Brown Univ., R.I. Hosp., Providence, RI, USA and
**CIBA-GEIGY Corp., Summit, NJ, USA

Erosion of articular cartilage is a hall mark of Osteoarthritis (OA). Articular cartilage is a unique tissue in that it is aneural, alymphatic, and avascular. Repair of "minor" damage to the tissue appears to be an ongoing process. On the other hand, "major" damage to the tissue seems to be irreversible. In contrast to many other tissues, biopsy of cartilage for diagnostic purposes cannot be justified.

To date, treatment has been limited largely to drugs which provide symptomatic relief of pain and inflammation, primarily non-steroidal anti-inflammatory drugs which act principally by inhibiting prostaglandin synthesis. The drugs of the future must either prevent loss of the connective tissues from cartilage and/or enhance the reparative processes of cartilage and not just be palliative.

Tests for detecting arthritic changes at the early stages of disease are not available. Consequently, present-day diagnosis relies on clinical manifestations or x-ray changes which can be observed only at later stages of disease progression. In the near future it is hoped that magnetic resonance imaging (MRI) of joints may be useful for the diagnosis of the early stages of OA. To overcome present-day limitations, biochemical markers have been sought in the synovial fluid or circulation. Since no therapy prevents progression of OA at this time, it is hoped that these markers can be used to monitor the effect of different treatment modalities.

Presentations at the Osteoarthritis Workshop of the 5th International Inflammation Research Association were focused on several different experimental approaches which could be used to induce

OA-like lesions in the knees of rabbits. Furthermore, the use of the rabbit knee as a system to monitor potential anti-OA drugs on connective tissue changes was explored and discussed.

Chelators Effect in vitro and in vivo

Collagen and proteoglycans, major constituents of the extracellular matrix of articular cartilage, are degraded by metalloproteinases e.g. collagenase, gelatinase and stromelysin. Several groups have demonstrated increased levels of activities of these enzymes in arthritic cartilage. Since these are divalent metal-dependent enzymes, it was hypothesized that the judicious use of metal-chelators may be appropriate therapy to inhibit cartilage erosion. Ehrlich and coworkers (Rhode Island Hosp.) found that EDTA (2 mM) given intraarticularly (i.a.) reduced neutral proteoglycanase of the cartilage by 25% and decreased disease severity in 75% of the rabbits in a surgical (Hulth-Telhag) model of OA. To ascertain whether reparative processes are maintained, they examined the effects of varying concentrations of EDTA and EGTA on cartilage integrity in both, "in vitro" and "in vivo" systems.

With the use of calf cartilage explants in an "in vitro" culture system, neither 1.5 mM EDTA nor 1.5 mM EGTA had any effect on total RNA or proteoglycan synthesis as reflected in ^{3}H-cytidine or ^{35}S-sulfate incorporation, respectively. However, 2 mM EDTA significantly inhibited both synthetic processes.

When examined "in vivo", this was not the case. Whereas 1.5 mM EGTA had no effect on RNA or proteoglycan synthesis when injected into the knees of mature New Zealand white rabbits, 2 mM EDTA caused a significant stimulation of both parameters. Of particular interest was the finding that with EDTA in 5 out of 6 normal rabbits, protease activity in the cartilage was inhibited between 14 and 60% when calf proteoglycan subunit was used as substrate. Thus, by both total RNA and proteoglycan synthesis, in vitro EDTA inhibited repair mechanisms whereas in vivo, an enhancement was indicated. These data, coupled to the apparent lack of adverse effects in this model, warrant further studies to examine a possible therapeutic role for metal chelators in the treatment of OA.

Plasminogen Activator in Rabbit Synovial Fluid after i.a. IL-1

Injections (i.a.) of recombinant human interleukin-1α (IL-1), shown previously to increase levels of degradative enzymes and to inhibit proteoglycan synthesis, has become a reproducible technique to initiate acute arthritic changes in animals. The IL-1 effects on connective tissue loss and enzyme levels as measured in the synovial fluid soon after initiation of the pathogenic process, could be useful parameters for drug screening.

Ganu and colleagues (Ciba-Geigy) evaluated cartilage degradation over a 54 h period by measuring levels of synovial fluid plasminogen activator (PA), synovial fluid keratan sulfate (KS), and the ratio of sulfated glycosaminoglycan to hydroxyproline (S-GAG/Hyp) in the rabbit knee cartilage after intra-articular injection of IL-1. The earliest detected change, an 8 to 10-fold elevation in PA activity, was followed by temporary increases in synovial fluid KS, and later by a decrease in cartilage S-GAG/Hyp ratio. since PA initiates a series of reactions which can result in the production of active stromelysin this model may be useful for evaluating suppressors of PA activity and consequently inhibitors of cartilage destruction. However, dexamethasone and indomethacin decreased the IL-1 induced increase in PA without protecting the cartilage from a loss of proteoglycans. Therefore, other mechanisms may be relevant in this model.

IL-1 and bFGF Synergism in Degrading Rabbit Cartilage in vivo

E. Shatzen and P. Stevens (Amgen) reported that basic fibroblast growth factor (bFGF) was found to potentiate the arthritic lesion produced by IL-1β when co-injected into rabbit knees. The synergistic effect of bFGF with IL-1 had previously been shown only in vitro. A single i.a. injection of IL-1β (10 kU) and bFGF (10 μg) resulted in a sustained and significant loss of proteoglycans over a 21 day period which was reflected in higher S-GAG contents in the synovial fluid. The synovial levels of proteoglycan constituents could be a useful system to evaluate not only potential anti-arthritic agents which interfere with proteoglycan catabolism, but also factors that may promote cartilage repair.

When injected alone, IL-1β caused relatively little loss of proteoglycans in the cartilage of the tibial plateau. This is in contrast to previous reports from other laboratories which demonstrated severe loss of proteoglycan from the femoral condyles after IL-1 (i.a.) treatment. The reason for the greater sensitivity to the actions of IL-1β in the latter site is unclear, although, it may be related inversely to the thickness of the cartilage. These data again emphasize the need to specify the anatomic site under consideration. For example, in surgically induced models of OA, maximal cartilage erosion is noted initially on the tibial plateau but later the femoral cartilage also sustains significant loss.

Continuous Infusion of IL-1 or Collagenase into Rabbit Knee

Borella and coworkers (Wyeth-Ayerst) used an Alzet osmotic pump, implanted subcutaneously, with a catheter situated in the synovial space of the rabbit knee to introduce either activated human collagenase (60 U/ml, from human skin fibroblast cultures) or recombinant IL-1β (40 to 2000 U/ml). IL-1β or the activated collagenase (7 days at a rate of 10 μl/h) induced cartilage damage in the joint as assessed by histology. Significant loss of proteoglycans and cell death were observed at the end of the experimental period. Synovitis was seen in both treatment groups.

Although this appears to be an attractive model in which to introduce and examine the effects of potential therapeutic agents, there was some caution expressed over possible non-specific cartilage damage resulting from accumulation of fluid in the intra-articular space. In addition, since these are preliminary studies, no data on progression or reversibility of cartilage damage was presented.

MRI of Cartilage in Rabbit Joints

Effective mechanisms for non-invasive monitoring of arthritic changes are being sought not only for diagnostic purposes, but also as means of evaluating therapeutic agents. O'Byrne and coworkers (CIBA-GEIGY and Laurie Imaging Center) used MRI to assess cartilage thickness in the knees of rabbits which had been subjected to i.a. injections of papain (5 U). This enzyme treatment is known to cause rapid loss of matrix constituents without fibrillation. Mean cartilage thickness was 1.08 $\pm$ 0.09 mm prior to papain injection (T2 images of femoral cartilage). A 35% loss in cartilage thickness was noted 24 h after papain treatment. This was accompanied by a 93% loss in proteoglycan content when measured with the dimethylmethylene blue dye binding assay. A 30% recovery in proteoglycan content as well as a 10% recovery of cartilage thickness was noted over the next 48 h.

Differences in scans because of alteration in water content resulting largely from loss of proteoglycans makes interpretation of the MRI scans difficult. Even though there is a decrease in proteoglycan content of cartilage there is also an increase of water content in early OA. The use of imaging for phosphorous or sodium instead of hydrogen may increase the specificity and sensitivity of this technique.

In summary, these presentations, based on rabbit knee model systems, suggest that MRI and synovial fluid markers may be useful parameters to evaluate cartilage alterations associated with the pathogenesis of OA.

AAS 35
Progress in Inflammation
Research and Therapy

C. Gordon Van Arman Scholarship Competition

R. P. Carlson and A. J. Lewis

Wyeth-Ayerst Research, Princeton, NJ 08543-8000, USA

The Inflammation Research Association sponsored a competition to encourage exploratory and applied research in inflammation among graduate students and post-doctoral fellows. Twelve researchers entered the second biennial competition for the C. Gordon Van Arman Awards at the 5th International Conference at White Haven, PA on September 23–27, 1990.

The awards have been named to recognize the example of C. Gordon Van Arman who has had a long research and distinguished career as an industrial scientist during which he published over 100 scientific papers. The development of the drugs diphenoxylate, disopyramide, sulindac, and diflunisal can be directly attributed to his work. In 1970, Dr. Van Arman with Edward I. Takesue, Marvin E. Rosenthale and Mary Lee Graeme founded the Inflammation Research Association as an informal forum for bench scientists to exchange research ideas in inflammatory diseases. By establishing this award, we wish to develop a commitment to high quality inflammation research in young scientists.

The Scholarship Committee selected the award winners based on a poster presentation to the committee (50%), a mini-paper (25%) and oral presentation (25%). All finalists received a travel grant of \$500 and the prizes of \$1000 (1st), \$500 (2nd), \$250 (3rd) and \$100 (honorable mention) were presented by Drs. Lewis and Carlson at the Conference Banquet.

The winners were:
1st place: Chean Eng Ooi, New York University School of Medicine, New York, NY.
2nd place: Keren I. Hulkower, Pittsburgh University School of Medicine, Pittsburgh, PA.
3rd Place: Helen Wheeler-Aceto, Temple University School of Medicine, Philadelphia, PA.
Honorable Mentions: Geethani Bandara, Pittsburgh University School of Medicine, Pittsburgh, PA; Chaman L. Chander, St. Bartholomew's Hospital Medical College, London, England; John Pawlowski, Pennsylavania University School of Medicine, Philadelphia, PA; and Amy H. Schultheis, The Johns Hopkins University, School of Hygiene and Public Health, Baltimore, MD.

The Van Arman Award participants added a refreshing and scholarly dimension to the Conference and we look forward to future award competitions.

Scholarship Committee:

Co-chairmans:	R. P. Carlson	A. J. Lewis
Members:	J. L. Humes	R. B. Gilbertsen
	M. J. DiMartino	I. G. Otterness
	R. J. Smith	

The following winning abstracts of the Gordon Van Arman Scholarship Competition will be reported in great detail as mini papers to be published in Agents and Actions in 1991 in a special issue on The 5th International Conference of the Inflammation Research Association at White Haven, PA.

Structural and Functional Organization of the Human Neutrophil 60 kDa Bactericidal/Permeability Protein

Chean Eng Ooi

Chean Eng Ooi presented studies on the purified bactericidal/permeability increasing protein (BPI) from human PMN which is bactericidal for several strains of gram negative bacteria. Studies of other toxins, including multifunctional and plant cytotoxins, have revealed that binding and catalytic functions are found on separate domains, although both domains are required for expression of cytotoxic activity. The 60 kDa BPI molecule could be proteolytically cleaved and separated into N- and C- terminal fragments. The NH_2-terminal amino acid sequence of purified fragments were determined by sequential Edman degradation using an automated sequentor (Beckman 890 or Applied Biosystems 470A) and was found to be more basic and less hydropholic than the holo-protein. The 25 kDa N-terminal fragment which is more hydrophobic than the C-terminal portion of BPI displayed full functional activity of BPI on a molar basis while the 30 kDa C-terminal fragment had no detectable antibacterial activity. Also, the 25 kDa fragment retains the specificity of BPI toward gram-negative bacteria. Ooi speculated that after PMN ingestion of bacteria an intracellular proteolytic event occurs which allows the hydropholic N-terminal fragment of BPI to bind tightly with the phagolysosome. These results imply a novel structural and functional organization of this specific cytotoxic protein, BPI.

Interleukin-1 and Synovial Protein Kinase C: Identification of a Novel, 35 kDa Cystosolic Substrate

Keren I. Hulkower

Keren Hulkower investigated the role of PKC in IL-1 activated lapine synovial fibroblasts. Whereas standard methods for assaying PKC activity failed to detect this enzyme in cellular fractions of synoviocytes, Western blotting revealed PKC activity in the cytosolic and membrane fractions of PMA activated cells. PMA has been reported to stimulate the redistribution (translocation) of PKC from a cystolic to a cell membrane domain in numerous cell types, and PKC redistribution was observed in PMA-activated synoviocytes. A 35 kDa protein, rather than the well established 80 kDa protein (not seen in lapine synovial cells), was found by Dr. Hulkower to be a major PKC substrate in synovial fibroblasts, and PMA stimulated the phosphorylation of this 35 kDa protein. Furthermore, protein kinase inhibitors such as staurosporine and H-7 suppressed neutral metalloproteinases (NMP) and prostanoid production by synoviocytes activated with PMA. Using monoclonal antibodies to PKC subspecies, Dr. Hulkower identified the α (type III) and β (type II) isozymes of PKC in synovial fibroblasts. Whether or not PKC isozymes catalyze the phosphorylation of cytosolic proteins in a function-specific manner and whether or not these PKC subspecies are activated in a stimulus-specific fashion remain open questions. In contrast to PMA, IL-1 stimulated neither PKC redistribution nor phosphorylation of the 35 kDa protein in synovial fibroblasts. In addition, protein kinase inhibitors had no effect on IL-1-stimulated NMP production by synoviocytes. The existence of an endogenous correlate of PMA notwithstanding, these data suggest that the responsiveness of synovial fibroblasts to IL-1, and quite possibly other cytokines, might be regulated by PKC-dependent and PKC-independent pathways. Thus, the results of these studies may provide insight to the mechanisms of cytokine-triggered tissue-degrading NMP production by synovial cells in inflammatory joint disease.

Neurogenic and Tissue-Mediated Components of Formalin-Induced Edema: Evidence for Supraspinal Regulation

Helen Wheeler-Aceto

Injection of formalin into the rat hind paw produces both localized pain and inflammation. The nociceptive effect of formalin, recorded as flinching/ shaking of the paw, is biphasic. Helen Wheeler-Aceto undertook a systematic investigation of the relationship between the formalin-induced pain and edema responses. The intent was to establish whether pain is involved in the initiation and development of edema and whether down-regulatory supraspinal inputs in fluenced both nociception and edema/inflammation. The edema (inflammatory response) to formalin is also biphasic. The rapid initiation of edema is associated with early phase nociception and is dependent on activity in primary afferent neurons and axon reflexes. Early edema (0–5 h) is reduced by peripheral nerve section and capsaicin treatment of the sciatic nerve. However, the late phase edema is potentiated at 24 h only by nerve section suggesting that persistent reflex activity in the absence of descending inhibition enhances inflammation. The overall findings indicate that formalin-induced edema results from a balance between afferent and efferent neuron activity. A supraspinal mechanism is responsible for regulating the inflammatory response. The identity of a putative anti-inflammatory substance is unknown although centrally released opioid peptides and corticotropin-releasing factor are potential candidates. These data supported this model to investigate the relationship between pain and inflammation. Moreover, peripheral and spinal targets for therapeutic modulation may be assessed using this model.

The Synovial Activation of Chondrocytes: Evidence for Complex Cytokine Interactions

Geethani Bandara

It is well established that synovial fibroblasts can secrete interleukin-1 (IL-1), which is felt to mediate a number of proinflammatory and tissue-destructive processes, including the production of neutral metalloproteinases (NMP) from chondrocytes. Bandara's investigations sought to determine if there were pro-inflammatory factors in addition to IL-1 which were produced by synovial fibroblasts. To answer this question, the HIG-82 line of rabbit synovial fibroblasts was examined for mRNA to various cytokines, and used as a source of chondrocyte activating factors (CAF) which were assayed for the ability to induce NMP production from confluent rabbit chondrocytes. Using Northern blot analysis, synovial fibroblasts were found to contain mRNA for TGFβ, basic fibroblast growth factor (bFGF), TNFα, and trace amounts of IL-6, in addition to message for IL-1β. CAF preparations contained IL-1, bFGF, TNFα, and trace amounts of IL-6. CAF stimulated NMP production more effectively than did either IL-1α or IL-1β, however, while purified TNFα and IL-6 were inactive. Using the interleukin-1 receptor antagonist protein (IRAP) obtained from Synergen, Bandara found that IRAP completely blocked NMP production induced by IL-1, but only partially blocked NMP production induced by CAF. These results collectively suggest that there may be factors, in addition to IL-1, but distinct from TNFα and IL-6, which are able to induce NMP production from rabbit chondrocytes.

The Effects of Estrogens on Cartilage Degradation Using *In Vivo* and *In Vitro* Models

Chaman L. Chander

Sex hormones have been proposed to influence the pathogenesis of osteoarthritis. However, their pharmacological effects in animal models of arthritis are complex and, often controversial. Thus, Chaman L. Chander attempted to clarify the role of 17β-estradiol in arthritic conditions by investigating its effect on cartilage degradation in *in vivo* and *in vitro* model systems. In the *in vivo* model, Chander implanted rat femoral head cartilage (FHC) subcutaneously into female mice. Prior to implantation, the FHC was wrapped in cotton in order to provoke granulomatous tissue and cartilage degradation, which was assessed by loss of glycosaminoglycans (GAGs). The administration of estradiol at 1 mg/kg/day s.c. for 14 days was found to accelerate GAG loss in FHC. Moreover, the administration of tamoxifen (4 and 8 mg/kg/day, p.o.), an anti-estrogen compound, reduced the degree of cartilage damage in a dose dependent manner. In *in vitro* studies, estradiol (10 μg/ml) was also found to induce loss of GAGs from FHC, in the presence or absence of fibroblasts. Although the doses of estradiol utilized in these studies were high and non-physiological, the results suggest that estrogen receptors may be involved in estradiol induced cartilage degradation, which is mediated by either a direct action on chondrocytes or through activation of fibroblasts. Chander demonstrated that estradiol, in pharmacological doses, accelerates cartilage degradation *in vivo* and *in vitro*. The physiological significance and implications of these findings require further study.

Isolation and Partial Characterization of a Full-Length cDNA Clone for 3α-Hydroxysteroid Dehydrogenase: A Potential Target Enzyme for Nonsteroidal Antiinflammatory Drugs

John Pawlowski

John Pawloski utilized a previous discovery in the same laboratory by Dr. T. M. Penning that nonsteroidal antiinflammatory drugs were potent inhibitors of 3α-hydroxysteroid dehydrogenase (3α-HSD) obtained from rat liver cytosol. This cytosolic enzyme binds arachidonic acid and prostaglandins at its active site and is inhibited by nonsteroidal antiinflammatory drugs in rank order of their therapeutic potency. A nonspecific, polyclonal anti-sera raised against the purified enzymes was used to screen a lgtll expression library and oligonucleotide probes complementary to the 5′ and 3′ ends of immunopositive clones were used to isolate a 2.1 Kb full-length cDNA. Digestion of the full-length cDNA generated a 1.1 Kb fragment containing the C-terminus of 3α-HSD. This C-terminus portion of 3α-HSD was sequenced and it demonstrated a significant homology (i.e. 53% at the nucleotide level and 71% at the amino acid level) to prostaglandin $F_2\alpha$ synthase isolated from bovine lung. These observations suggest that 3α-HSD and prostaglandin synthase are members of a common gene family. In addition, these data may implicate a role for 3α-HSD in inflammation.

Inflammatory Cell Influx Into Ozone-Exposed Guinea Pig Lung Interstitial and Airway Spaces

Amy H. Schultheis

Amy Schultheis evaluated a model of non-immunological lung inflammation, whereby guinea pigs were exposed to 2.0 ppm ozone for 4 hours. At 0 time (4 h after ozone exposure) neutrophils had accumulated to >4 times control in the lung interstitium but declined to control values 24 h. Bronchoalveolar lavage (BAL) recovered neutrophils were maximum by 3–4 h and remained elevated for 3 days post ozone. Macrophage numbers were doubled in lavageable spaces at 2 days but declined to normal at day 7 while macrophages in the interstitium increased by only a third and remained elevated through 14 days. Eosinophils were significantly elevated at 3 days in the BALF of the ozone treated guinea pigs and decreased below control values (post exposure) at day 14. Total lymphocyte counts were unaltered during the course of the experiment. This model of ozone-induced lung inflammation does not distinguish in the lung digest between inflammatory cells adhering to endothelium or those that infiltrated into the interstitium. BAL measurements may not necessarily reflect the initial inflammatory response within the lung since the lung digest total neutrophil count peaked at 0 time (4 h post-ozone) compared to the BAL peak counts at 3–4 h which remained elevated for several days (i.e. chronic inflammation). Interestingly, the high interstitial neutrophilic count initially may be due to these cells sticking to the endothelial cells right after the ozone exposure and being released later into the circulation. Macrophage accumulation in the BAL at 2 to 3 days may be due to ozone damage to the terminal broncholar ciliated cells which are involved in transport of macrophages out of the lung.

Poster Discussion

AAS 35
Progress in Inflammation
Research and Therapy

Autoimmunity Poster Discussion Group

Co-Chairmen: N. D. Staite and R. B. Gilbertsen***

*The Upjohn Co., Kalamazoo, MI 49002
**Parke-Davis Pharm. Res. Ann Arbor, MI 48105

Nine posters were presented in this session, which was divided into three broad topics, each containing three presentations. Following the display of posters, the presenters were asked to give brief summations of their work, and a discussion was held at the end of each topic.

Rapamycin in Models of Autoimmunity and Transplantation

W. L. Baeder (Wyeth-Ayerst) showed that rapamycin, given to non-obese diabetic (NOD/Mrk) female mice, can prevent the development of diabetes mellitus. Onset of diabetes was determined when plasma glucose exceeded 200 mg/dL and greater than 70% of untreated animals are normally diabetic by 20–25 weeks of age. Rapamycin, in a vehicle of 8% cremophor/2% ethanol, was given orally, three times a week, from 56 days of age. Rapamycin at 6 and 12 mg/kg prevented the onset of diabetes as evidenced by a normal plasma glucose level (149 ± 5 mg/dL) compared with untreated animals (475 ± 69 mg/dL). Cyclosporin-A (12 mg/kg), however, was ineffective in this model with mice developing plasma glucose levels of 562 ± 52 mg/dL. During discussion it was pointed out that ineffectiveness of cyclosporin-A may be the result of the dose used, although cyclosporin-A is active at 12–15 mg/kg in other models (e.g., adjuvant arthritis).

L. Warner (Wyeth-Ayerst) also addressed the immunosuppressive activity of rapamycin in a host vs. graft popliteal lymph node proliferation assay which is driven by an *in vivo* mixed lymphocyte reaction. Recipient mice (C3H, H-2^k) were injected with irradiated CTLL-2 cells (H-2^b) into one paw and popliteal lymph node proliferation, associated with the injected paw, measured by *in vivo* tritiated thymidine uptake. Rapamycin given orally at 6 μg/kg-6 mg/kg suppressed lymph node proliferation by 33 ± 7 to $76 \pm 5\%$. Intraperitoneal administration produced greater inhibition at the lower doses. Cyclosporin-A (60 μg/kg-6 mg/kg) given orally or intraperitoneally was less effective (40 ± 10 to $24 \pm 6\%$ suppression).

E. O. Ohia (Univ. of Louisville) showed that rapamycin, cyclosporin-A, and topical corticosteroid were immunosuppressive in a heterolamellar corneal transplant model. Bovine corneal lamella was transplanted onto the cornea of rabbits, which typically results in conjuctival hyperemia and edema for 3–5 days, followed by angiogenesis and graft rejection within 7–10 days. Rapamycin (1 mg/kg) and cyclosporin-A (25 mg/kg), given intramuscularly once a day, inhibited the hyperemia and edema seen after surgery, as well as the angiogenic and delayed-type hypersensitivity responses. Grafts survived for 20 days, but when treatment was stopped (day 20), rejection took place on days 28 and 25, respectively. Topical dexamethasone (0.1%) or prednisolone (1%), given three times a day, not only inhibited rejection up to day 20 but prevented graft rejection until day 55, once treatment was stopped on day 20. Together with previous studies in MRL/lpr mice and collagenase-induced arthritis, these three presentations provide additional animal data that rapamycin is an effective immunosuppressive agent.

Immunosuppressive Agents in Models of SLE and EAE

This series of presentations focused on the effects of leflunomide (HWA 486) and 15-deoxyspergualin (15-DOS) on MRL/lpr mice and experimental allergic encephalomyelitis (EAE) in rats. R. R. Bartlett (Hoechst AG) presented a comparative study of leflunomide and cyclosporin-A in the treatment of MRL/lpr mice. Both agents suppressed the lymphadenopathy resulting from the proliferation of

Thy1$^+$, CD3$^+$, CD5$^+$, B220$^+$, CD4$^-$, CD8$^-$ T-cells and normalized the abnormally high ratio of CD4 : CD8 cells. The total number of CD4$^+$ cells was suppressed by cyclosporin-A and less so by leflunomide. Leflunomide, however, suppressed proteinuria while cyclosporin-A only delayed its onset. This may be related to the more suppressive effect of leflunomide on levels of circulating immune complexes and anti-DNA antibodies. Leflunomide is a prodrug which undergoes a ring-opening reaction. It is currently undergoing clinical trials in patients with rheumatoid arthritis at 5, 10, and 25 mg/day, with promising early data at the 25 mg/day dose. Data on leflunomide was presented at the 4th IRA meeting in 1988 suggesting it primarily inhibits Th2, T-helper cells. Recent evidence suggests it may be a tyrosine kinase inhibitor.

H. U. Schorlemmer (Behringwerke) gave two posters on the anti-proliferative agent, 15-DOS. Treatment of MRL/lpr mice with 5 mg/kg 15-DOS decreased anti-DNA and anti-collagen antibody levels. Proteinuria and glomerular nephritis were also suppressed leading to an overall improvement in survival rate in 15-DOS treated animals. 15-DOS also appeared to be effective in the treatment of established disease. In acute EAE in rats, which leads to death by day 15, 15-DOS reduced paralysis and deaths as well and preventing subsequent relapses. Treated animals were also resistant to re-challenge with guinea pig spinal cord. In a chronic, relapsing EAE model using myelin basic protein, 15-DOS treated animals survived the first disease episode and did not develop secondary of tertiary relapses, as were seen in control animals. 15-DOS may suppress B-lymphocytes more than T-lymphocytes which would suggest that it would be useful in controlling autoantibody production. The utility of 15-DOS will depend on its toxicity profile. One study has reported that 15-DOS could cause intestinal lesions and bone marrow toxicity which would be consistent with its anti-proliferative mechanism of action.

Regulation of Autoimmune Responses

H. U. Schorlemmer described the effects of an anti-rat α/β T-cell receptor antibody (R73) on adjuvant arthritis, EAE, and a graft vs.

host popliteal lymph node assay. R73 (0.5 mg) given on days 1–3 and 12–14 suppressed adjuvant arthritis. Antibody treatment was more effective if given from the time of induction of arthritis compared with established disease. R73 also suppressed EAE and reduced popliteal lymph node proliferation in the *in vivo* MLR assay. These findings are in agreement with a growing number of human clinical trials in which some anti-CD3, CD4, and CD5 antibodies are proving effective in the treatment of rheumatoid arthritis.

L. van de Langerijt (Univ. Nijmegen) showed that T-cells, isolated from Lewis rats with adjuvant arthritis, can passively transfer disease to normal Lewis but not the resistant Fisher strain 344. Correspondingly, *in vitro* proliferative responses to mycobacterial antigen were present in spleen and lymph node cells from recipient Lewis but not F344 rats. Cell mixing experiments suggested that F344 rats had a population of suppressor cells that prevented passive transfer of arthritis. Since germ-free F344 rats are susceptible to the induction of adjuvant or streptococcal cell wall arthritis, it is possible that these suppressor cells may develop after exposure to bacterial antigens present on gut flora.

M. van Bruggen (Univ. Nijmegen) presented complimentary studies on the transfer of streptococcal cell wall (SCW) arthritis in Lewis (susceptible) and F344 (resistant) rats. Transplantation of bone marrow from F344 to irradiated Lewis rats converted the recipients into SCW resistant animals. Conversely, bone marrow chimeras produced by transfer of Lewis bone marrow into F344 rats rendered these animals susceptible to arthritis. Similar results were obtained when adjuvant-induced arthritis was induced in the respective chimeras. This suggests that resistance of F344 rats to both forms of experimentally-induced arthritis is linked to stem cells in the marrow.

Both co-chairmen would like to extend their thanks to the presenters and participants in this session for making the autoimmunity poster discussion group a success.

AAS 35
Progress in Inflammation
Research and Therapy

Phospholipase A_2 Poster Discussion Session

L. A. Marshall and K. M. Tramposch

SmithKline Beecham Pharmaceuticals, King of Prussia, PA 19406, USA and Bristol-Myers Squibb, Buffalo, NY 14213, USA

The Poster-Discussion Session on phospholipase A_2 (PLA_2) focused on two important questions which have pre-occupied those interested in developing selective PLA_2 inhibitors. First, which PLA_2-type activity is the appropriate target for development of an anti-inflammatory agent? Second, which pharmacological models are most appropriate for the assessment of PLA_2 inhibitors? Ten posters were chosen which addressed these questions either directly or indirectly, or contributed information toward discussion of the questions.

Which PLA_2-Type Activity is the Appropriate Target for Development of an Anti-Inflammatory Drug?

Phospholipase A_2 plays a key role in the production of lipid inflammatory mediators, e.g., prostaglandins (PGs), leukotrienes (LTs), platelet activating factor (PAF) and, therefore, has been selected as a pharmacological target for development of novel anti-inflammatory agents. Since the success of both molecular modeling and creative drug design efforts depends directly on the relevance of the biological assay system, selection of the appropriate enzyme target is critical. A number of PLA_2 enzymes have been described and utilized for compound evaluation including non-mammalian, mammalian and human-derived enzymes. PLA_2-like activity is found in a variety of tissues and plays an important role in normal cell lipid maintenance and lipid mediator formation. Additionally, PLA_2 also plays other physiological roles including enzymatic digestion. A new functional role was proposed by M. Fry et al. (Virginia Commonwealth University, Richmond, VA) who described a sn-2 acylhydrolytic activity found in human sperm. The sperm enzyme is a low MW (12 kDa), Ca^{++} requiring enzyme. This enzyme may participate in sperm penetration into the oocyte and therefore contribute to the induction of fertilization. They showed that blockade of this enzyme by the prostaglandin polymer PGBx could dose-dependently block sperm penetration of hamster oocytes.

Acylhydrolytic enzymes appear both intra- and extracellularly, some soluble and others associated with membrane fractions. It is therefore not surprising that PLA_2s have been reported to be biochemically and structurally distinct. Sn-2 acylhydrolytic enzymes, so far described vary in molecular weight, in their requirement for calcium and in the sn-2 acyl group specificity. Since species structural heterogeneity exists and the effect of this on catalysis and inhibitory selectivity is not yet defined, human enzymes may prove to be the most relevant choice as drug targets. L. Marshall et al. (SmithKline Beecham, PA) reviewed the biochemical profile of two human enzymes, i.e., a soluble 14 kDa PLA_2 isolated from the joint fluid of patients with inflammatory joint disease and an intracellular cytosolic 110 kDa PLA_2 isolated from a human monocytic cell line, U-937. The high molecular weight enzyme primarily differed from the low molecular weight PLA_2 in its lower (nM) Ca^{++} requirement and its preference for arachidonic acid (AA) in the sn-2 position of phospholipid substrate. Pharmacological evaluation of the two enzymes revealed that a phosphonate-phospholipid analogue was 100-fold more effective against the low molecular weight than the high molecular weight, suggesting that the two enzymes were catalytically distinct and could be selectively regulated by pharmacological agents. J. S. Kerr et al. (E. I. du Pont de Nemours & Co. Inc., Wilmington, DE) described their purification of a low molecular weight 17 kDA PLA_2 isolated from the membrane of U-937 cells which demonstrated a preference for 1-0-alkyl-containing phospholipid (PL). This enzyme was not isolated using the often used acid extraction procedure but rather purified through a series of chromatographic techniques indicating that the isolation procedure chosen could mask or destroy important PLA_2 isotypes which may potentially contribute to cellular lipid metabolism.

Whereas, our knowledge of human PLA_2 enzymes is expanding, the question remains whether or not one should target cell-associated enzymes or the so called "secreted" or soluble low MW PLA_2 found in inflammatory exudate for drug development? Little is known about the source and/or mechanism of activation of the soluble PLA_2 activity which is enhanced in serum or tissue fluids during an inflammatory episode. This was addressed by Goodman et al. (E. I. du Pont De Nemours & Co. Inc., Wilmington, DE) showing that human recombinant IL-1β and TNF-α affect PLA_2 activity in bovine pulmonary artery endothelial cells and induce its release into surrounding media. This suggested that cytokine production during inflammation could propagate the disease state through release of extracellular acylhydrolytic activity and concomitant eicosanoid production.

Other sn-2 hydrolyzing enzymes such as acyltransferases have been described. These enzymes co-exist with classical PLA_2 enzymes and may influence the activity of PLA_2 and/or contribute directly to lipid mediator formation. One such enzyme, CoA-independent transacylase, was characterized by J. Winkler et al. (SmithKline Beecham, King of Prussia, PA). This enzyme selectively transfers arachidonic acid from the sn-2 position of diacylphospholipids to the sn-2 position of 1-0-alkyl-containing lyso phospholipids. In so doing, this enzyme may control the substrate pool used for formation of PAF. CoA-IT was distinct from classical PLA_2 since it was Ca^{++}-independent, strongly membrane-associated, heat and acid unstable and not responsive to classical PLA_2 modifiers such as dexamethasone, aristolochic acid or arachidonic acid.

Taken together, the enzymes described may make up only a fraction of the sn-2 acylhydrolytic activity that actually exist. This therefore makes it difficult to choose the most appropriate target enzyme for drug screening. It is clear that much more work must be done to delineate the "pro-inflammatory" PLA_2 which is to be pharmacologically modified in an effort to control the initiation and/or propagation of inflammation. Nonetheless, the biochemical differences described between the low molecular weight PLA_2 isotypes, high molecular weight PLA_2 and various transacylases are encouraging in that inhibitor selectivity may be possible when designing novel PLA_2 inhibitors. Selective inhibitors of PLA_2 would minimize potential liabilities or side effects resulting from global lipase inhibition.

Which Pharmacological Model is most Appropriate to Assess PLA_2 Inhibitors?

Once biochemically-defined PLA_2 inhibitors are identified, they must be tested *in vivo* to establish drug efficacy. Whereas information is slowly becoming available on the types of human PLA_2 that exist, there is a paucity of information on differentiation between PLA_2 basal activity and enhancement of this activity which may or may not be expressed during an inflammatory insult. Can models be developed or do models currently exist that could differentiate between these two activity levels? The lack of an orally active selective PLA_2 inhibitor makes resolution of this issue more difficult.

One approach taken is to biochemically assess the effects of PLA_2 by measuring lipid mediator production. This can be performed *in vitro* using stimulated cell populations or *in vivo* by evaluating the mediators present in exudate fluids retrieved from various animal models. K. Glaser et al. (Wyeth-Ayerst Research, Princeton, NJ) described the effects of putative PLA_2 and 5-LO inhibitors on the biosynthesis of PAF and LTB_4 by A23187-induced human PMN. One PLA_2 inhibitor, luffariellolide, dose-dependently blocked PAF production. Inhibitors of LTB_4 biosynthesis such as Wy 50295 and A-64077 had no effect on PAF formation. L-663,536, a 5-LO translocation inhibitor, blocked both LTB_4 and at higher concentrations blocked PAF production. The inhibition of PAF by L-663,536 exemplifies an issue which should be considered when cellular assays are used to evaluate effects on PLA_2 via mediator release. These types of assays are sensitive to agents which can affect non-PLA_2 enzymes and block the mediator in question and it is important to completely evaluate the mechanism and selectivity of putative PLA_2 inhibitors.

G. W. DeVries et al. (Allergen Inc./Herbert Laboratories, Irvine, CA) demonstrated that AGN 190383, a 2(5H)-furanone ring analogue of manoalide, inhibited AA released from human PMN exposed to A23187 ($IC_{50} = 0.8\ \mu M$) and they proposed that this could account, in part, for the anti-inflammatory action observed when the drug was topically applied to mouse ears exposed to phorbol ester. They demonstrated a positive correlation between AGN 190383 inhibition *in vitro* and an *in vivo* inflammatory response, the reduction in inflammatory ear edema. While this data was encouraging, it was not conclusive since the drug displayed a lack of selectivity through its activity against another cellular lipase, PLC. This enzyme as well as other lipases (e.g., PLD) not examined, may contribute to activated-release of free fatty acid and potentially affect the interpretation of the mechanism by which AGN 190383 produces *in vivo* anti-inflammatory activity.

Two major approaches have been utilized in deciding which model to use for whole animal assessment of PLA_2 inhibitor action. One such route is to evaluate PLA_2 inhibitor efficacy in established models of inflammation. An example was described by C.E.T. Bak et al. (Hoffman-LaRoche Inc., Nutley, NJ) where eicosanoid production and elicited-peritoneal macrophage PLA_2 was assessed in adjuvant-arthritic rats. Direct evidence for enhanced cellular PLA_2 enzymatic activity due to the disease state was not found. However, PGE_2 production was 2-fold greater than that obtained from control rats supporting a major role for PGE_2 in the etiology of this model. This study typifies a model where clinical and biochemical measurements could be obtained to assess the effects of PLA_2 inhibitors. A cautionary note was revealed during the discussion suggesting that removal and washing of cells from drug-dosed animals could locally remove the drug and in cases of reversibility, abrogate the actual effects of the drug. L. D. Faison et al. (Wellcome Research Laboratory, Research Triangle Park, NC) presented another model where both LTB_4 and PAF could be directly assessed in the pleurisy fluid of rats pre-injected with the phlogistic agent, zymosan. Again, these lipid mediators could be examined in conjunction with clinical markers such as cellular infiltration or fluid accumulation.

New model development is the second route investigators have sought to define PLA_2 inhibitor action in the whole animal. One such model described by D. Hartmann et al. (Wyeth-Ayerst Research, Princeton, NJ) was the induction of mouse paw edema by the direct injection of isolated snake venom PLA_2 (D-49 A.p.p.). Interestingly, this model is primarily mediated via histamine release in addition to eicosanoid generation. Dexamethasone was a weak inhibitor at best while scalaradial, a PLA_2 inhibitor identified by R. Jacobs (Marine Science Institute, UCSB, Santa Barbara, CA), proved effective in reducing edema. A criticism was raised concerning the appropriateness of this model since it was snake venom PLA_2. This concern is magnified if the primary screens used to identify test compounds utilizes a human-derived enzyme. We must view this model as prototypical and useful in defining the pro-inflammatory effect of PLA_2. Human enzyme is currently not available in large quantities and until this tool is provided potential for false negatives using this approach could be high.

Several other examples of both established and newly developed models exist and are currently under evaluation for use in testing PLA_2 inhibitors. The choice of models is wide and varied due to the potential broad spectrum effects of lipid mediator modulation in a variety of tissues. The final assessment of model appropriateness must wait for the identification of an *in vivo* active, selective PLA_2 inhibitor.

The PLA_2 poster discussion session was a valuable one in that it clearly demonstrated that this area of research is maturing. Researchers are now beginning to focus on specific isotypes of PLA_2s as enzyme targets and it seems clear that specific inhibitors will surely follow. Once compounds are identified we will be able to test the hypothesis that PLA_2 activity is important in the inflammatory reaction.

AAS 35
Progress in Inflammation
Research and Therapy

Inflammatory Cells – Posters and Presentations

J. S. Kerr and D. W. Morgan***

*The Du Pont Merck Pharmaceutical Co., Wilmington, DE 19880-0400, USA
**Hoffmann-La Roche Inc., Nutley, NJ 07110, USA

The recent workshop in conjunction with the 5th International Conference of the Inflammation Research Association reviewed some recent progress associated with inflammatory cells. The poster presentations were divided into two broad areas: Cellular Mechanisms in Inflammation and New Anti-Inflammatory Agents. In the Cellular Mechanisms in Inflammation section, a rabbit model of skin lesions produced by the topical application of sulfur mustard was described. The effects of stimulation of human neutrophils by granulocyte/macrophage colony stimulating factor (GM-CSF) and tumor necrosis factor alpha (TNF-α) on superoxide production and phosphatidylcholine breakdown by phospholipase D were presented. The functions of other cells participating in the inflammatory process were also presented, including the accumulation of eosinophils in polymixin B induced airway hyperreactivity, the effect of protein kinase inhibitors on stimulated ELAM-1 expression on endothelial cells, and macrophage-mediated killing of splenic lymphocytes in adjuvant-induced arthritis. In the new Anti-Inflammatory Agents section, the effects of Tenidap, and specific NSAIDs and DMARDs on leukotriene B_4 (LTB_4)-mediated human neutrophil chemotaxis were discussed. The actions of the LTB_4 receptor antagonist SC-41930 were also presented. The mechanisms of these drugs should lead to a more comprehensive understanding of the inflammatory process.

Cellular Mechanisms in Inflammation

A. M. Dannenberg, Jr. (Professor, Experimental Pathology, The Johns Hopkins University School of Hygiene and Public Health) presented an animal model in rabbits in which skin lesions were produced by topical application of sulfur mustard. The lesions were free from microorganisms, and were organ cultured at the peak stage (1 and 2 days) and at the healing stage of the lesions (6 and 10 days). The extracellular fluids within the lesions were also analyzed. Extravasated serum was the major modulator of the acute inflammation. This serum turned over 3x per day and contained extracellular proteases such as collagenase and proteoglycanase as well as the serum proteinase inhibitors α1-proteinase inhibitor and the α-macroglobulins. During healing, the proteinase inhibitors decreased, allowing the extracellular proteineases to begin remodeling. The major cell types involved in this acute non-septic inflammation were activated macrophages and fibroblasts. Granulocytes passed through these lesions to the surface and became part of the lesion's crust. This crust contained digestive enzymes and probably antimicrobial factors to protect the tissues from infection. Also the crust contained growth factors necessary for re-epithelialization. This model enables the investigation of an inflammatory process from its initiation through the healing process without the presence of microorganisms.

In the second discussion, F. Cerasoli (Hoffmann-La Roche Inc., Nutley, NJ) described the association of eosinophil accumulation and their enhanced function in a model of airway hyperreactivity induced by polymyxin B administration. Antigen challenge of sensitized guinea pigs is known to produce airway hyperreactivity, massive airway eosinophilia, and enhanced superoxide anion release from airway eosinophils. Dr. Cerasoli and his co-workers attempted to mimic these conditions using repeated, aerosolized polymyxin B sulfate exposure to induce airway eosinophilia. They found that 24 hours after as few as five daily exposures to polymyxin, airway eosinophilia increased eight-fold, airway hyperreactivity was present, and superoxide anion release from isolated airway eosinophils increased two to five-fold. These responses were present (with greater magnitude) 24 hours after 21 exposures; however, they reversed between 24 and 48 hours after the last exposure. As suggested by these findings, Dr. Cerasoli concluded that airway eosinophilia can be produced by antigen-independent means and that airway hyperreactivity, possible due to enhanced eosinophil function, is also present.

In the third discussion, R. M. Schultz (Lilly Research Laboratories, Indianapolis, IN) addressed the potential intracellular mechanisms underlying the rather profound effects of GM-CSF on human neutrophils. These effects include inhibition of neutrophil motility, degranulation, induction of CD11b surface adhesion molecules, and enhanced phagocytosis. Schultz and co-workers first sought to determine whether GM-CSF was capable of directly enhancing the oxidative metabolism of human neutrophils, under experimental conditions where neutrophils were allowed to adhere by a CD1/CD18-dependent mechanism to keyhole limpet hemocyanin (KLH). They found that recombinant human GM-CSF induced significant superoxide production in human neutrophils within 30 minutes after addition of stimulus, and that the response was complete within two hours. The time-course of superoxide release correlated with adherence to KLH. In contrast, CM-CSF failed to induce superoxide release under conditions where neutrophils were maintained in suspension. Shultz thought that prolonged adherence to surface during exposure to GM-CSF may possibly constitute an important control mechanism in the host.

To deduce which intracellular mechanisms may be functioning in the neutrophil responses to GM-CSF, Shultz used a panel of pharmacologic inhibitors (Rolipram, staurosporine and cytochalasin B) to compare GM-CSF-induced superoxide to that produced by cells exposed to fMet-Leu-Phe and 12 myristate 13-acetate. Schultz suggested that intact PK-C activity is essential for neutrophil superoxide production, but that differences exist in the initial pathways induced by these neutrophil activators. He concluded that superoxide secretion from GM-CSF-treated neutrophils appears to be a direct, delayed response that requires assembly of microfilaments during exposure to the cytokine. These findings may help in our understanding of the pharmacological activities of GM-CSF as this cytokine is applied clinically.

New Antiinflammatory Agents

In the first discussion, T. Gaginella (Searle Research and Development, Skokie, IL) indicated that there is substantial evidence to implicate LTB_4 as a major mediator in inflammatory responses in inflammatory bowel disease (IBD) and psoriasis. He cited studies which measured elevated levels of LTB_4 in IBD and psoriasis; he made the observation that drugs effective in treating these diseases have been shown to reduce tissue LTB_4 levels; and that oxygen radicals may also contribute to the pathophysiology of IBD. Dr. Gaginella emphasized the potential utility of SC-41930 for the treatment of IBD. Although initially identified as an LTB_4 receptor antagonist, SC-41930 is now known to exhibit a number of antiinflammatory activities including inhibition of oxygen radical formation by human neutrophils.

The *in vitro* spectrum of SC-41930 activity includes binding to human granulocyte LTB_4 receptors, antagonizing the chemotactic and degranulating activities of LTB_4 competitively and inhibiting the chemotactic and degranulating responses induced by fMet-Leu-Phe and C5a. In guinea pig lung homogenates, SC-41930 binds to LTD_4 receptor binding sites with activity much weaker than FPL-55712. *In vivo* studies indicated that SC-41930 blocks granulocyte chemotaxis into a site of intradermal LTB_4 injection in guinea pigs and pretreatment with approximately 20 mg/kg intrarectally or orally blocks the production of colitis induced by acetic acid in rodents. Studies on HL-60 cells indicate that SC-41930 blocks the production of LTB_4 and PGE_2; this also occurs in guinea pig skin, indicating that the drug may have some phospholipase A_2 inhibitory activity. Some 5-lipoxygenase inhibitory activity of the compound also has been observed in *in vitro* assays, but it is virtually inactive against sheep seminal vesicle cyclooxygenase.

Dr. Gaginella concluded saying that the profile of this agent indicates that it may be a useful antiinflammatory drug for different types of inflammation, most notably those affecting the distal intestinal and colonic mucosa and the skin. The efficacy of SC-41930 may possibly be accounted for by mechanisms in addition to LTB_4 receptor antagonism. It is hoped that successful clinical studies with this agent will lead to a new therapeutic to treat IBD.

In the second discussion, H. J. Showell (Department of Immunology and Infectious Diseases, Pfizer Central Research) presented evidence that inhibition of LTB – mediated chemotaxis in human neutrophils may be an important component of the pharmacologic profile of many currently employed anti-inflammatory agents, including Tenidap. However, this property may not be optimally expressed *in vivo*. Tenidap inhibited LTB_4-mediated chemotaxis by human neutrophils with an $IC_{50} = 6.6\ \mu M$. All NSAIDs tested (salicylates, acetic acids, proprionic acids, pyrozoles, oxicams) had this property, with IC_{50} values ranging from $34\ \mu M$ (meclofenamate) to ~ 2 mM (aspirin and salicylic). This characteristic was less consistent with the DMARDs tested, with gold sodium thiomalate active with an $IC_{50} = 8.3\ \mu M$, and sulfasalazine with an $IC_{50} = 34\ \mu M$. D-penicillamine, chloroquine, and cyclosporine A were inactive. These agents exhibited specificity for the effect on neutrophil chemotaxis. Tenidap is an interesting drug, the mechanism(s) of which continue to be elucidated.

AAS 35
Progress in Inflammation
Research and Therapy

Non-Rheumatic Inflammatory Diseases

R. R. Harris and B. M. Weichman***

*E.I. Du Pont de Nemours & Co., P.O. Box 80400, Wilmington, DE 19880-0400
and **Wyeth-Ayerst Research, CN–8000, Princeton, NJ 08543-8000

Introduction

The poster discussion on Non-Rheumatic Inflammatory Diseases was divided into two sections, posters dealing with gastrointestinal inflammatory diseases and ones on topics of skin inflammation, asthma, and autoimmune diseases.

Gastrointesinal Inflammatory Diseases

N. K. Clapp (Oak Ridge Associate Universities, Oak Ridge, TN) presented the first poster which profiled the cotton top tamarin colitis models both in the acute and chronic stages. Myeloperoxidase levels, PAF, and IL1-β were increased in the colons of these animals suggesting that IL1-β and PAF may play a role in this disease. In a similar finding, P. C. Will (Hoffmann-LaRoche, Inc., Nutley, NJ) presented data that PAF levels were increased in acetic acid induced colitis in rats, and WEB 2086 and RO 24-0238, two PAF antagonists, reduced the severity of the disease.

R. E. Walsh et al. (Searle Laboratories, Skokie, IL) presented data on the effects of SC-41930, a LTB_4 receptor antagonist, in the acetic acid induced colitis model. SC-41930 reduced the influx of PMNs as determined by myeloperoxidase. SC-41930 also reduced the levels of LTB_4, suggesting possible other actions of the drug.

D. Buckman (Hoffman-LaRoche, Inc., Nutley, NJ) presented evidence that bradykinin-induced electrolyte secretion was inhibited by lonapalene, a 5 lipoxygenase inhibitor. The authors suggested that mediators other than the prostaglandins may be responsible for the secretion observed.

M. J. S. Miller et al. (LSU School of Medicine, New Orleans, LA) provided data which suggested that *misoprostol*, a prostaglandin analogue, would attenuate the damage in a rabbit model of necrotizing enterocolitis suggesting that prostaglandins may play a role in this disease.

Taken together the above presentations suggested that PAF, histamine and leukotrienes may play a role in colitis, and that PAF antagonists or 5 lipoxygenase inhibitors may have utility in treating this disease.

Skin Inflammation, Asthma and Autoimmune Disease

R. R. Harris (Du Pont, Wilmington, DE) presented data on Brequinar, an antiproliferative, in a skin hyperplasia model which showed that, unlike methotrexate, Brequinar works topically. This molecule may offer a topical antiproliferative treatment for psoriasis. D. J. Fretland (Searle Laboratories, Skokie, IL) further characterized SC 41930, the LTB_4 antagonist, showing that it also had activity in various skin inflammation models.

D. Fretland's group also showed that SC 41930 had activity in experimental allergic encephalomyelitis in the guinea pig. These data suggest a possible role of LTB_4 in this animal model of multiple sclerosis.

C. DeHaas (ICI Americas, Wilmington, DE) presented data on a model of dyspnea where tachykinin is the mediator. Thiorphan shifted the dose response curve of tackykinin to the right. Compounds such as atropine or propranolol had no effect in this model.

S. Wong (Merrifield Laboratories) presented data which suggested that an extract from Oxalis corniculata had an anti-diabetic effect by stimulating the growth of Islets of langerhans in animals.